The Healing Power
of Coconut

Publications International, Ltd.

Written by Jacqueline B. Marcus, MS, RDN, LDN, CNS, FADA, FAND

Photography from Shutterstock.com

ISBN: 978-1-68022-842-7

Manufactured in China.

8 7 6 5 4 3 2 1

Table of Contents

Introduction

Most people wouldn't recognize the term *"Cocos nucifera."* But the fruit of the palm *Cocos nucifera*—the incredible coconut—is a multidimensional and tremendously useful member of the plant kingdom. It can help you to prevent and treat some common health problems, nourish your body and groom your hair and nails, supercharge your metabolism, and much more.

Coconuts provide concentrated energy in their "meat," refreshing hydration in their water, hardy fibers for household necessities like brushes and twine, and a hard shell that can be converted into charcoal or used for various handcraft applications—and all these uses come in one compact and economical package!

Coconut Origins

Coconut palms may have originated in Malaysia. This conclusion is based on the number of species of insects around the world that are associated with coconut palms, but botanists do not fully agree.

A broader viewpoint is that coconuts originated somewhere in tropical Asia. Part of what makes their origin so difficult to pinpoint is that coconuts are so hardy. It is speculated that coconut seeds probably floated to different parts of the globe before humans transported them to different cultures.

Some early evidence of coconut use comes from the Marquesans, who have lived on a group of small islands located in the south Pacific a few degrees south of the equator since around 300 AD. Coconuts were thought to been consumed in a variety of ways throughout the Marquesas. Immature coconuts were cut open and their creamy interiors were used to nourish children. Coconut "cream" was extracted from freshly grated coconut meat, which was also

The coconut has been a staple in the diet of many cultures for thousands of years, primarily growing between the fronds at the crown of large tree-like palms that exceed 100 feet in tropical climates.

combined into other dishes. Marquesan men grated coconuts with an apparatus that looked like a sawhorse. The coconut blossom was also a favorite food source. Its sap, called *jekamai,* was heated to prevent fermentation and the sweet syrup of the blossom was used to flavor dishes.

Europeans first recognized the existence of coconuts in the Middle Ages, though Arab traders might have introduced coconuts to Eastern Africa much earlier. The explorer Marco Polo, a Venetian explorer and merchant traveller who engaged in an epic round-trip Asian journey that lasted 24 years, is said to have discovered coconuts in Java and the Nicobar Islands in Southeast Asia.

While the coconut was reportedly mentioned in ancient eastern Indian documents, the Asian geography that is west of India is not truly suitable for its growth—nor is the south of China. Excursions by sailors and tradesmen both north and south brought coconuts into new lands.

During pre-Columbian times in Central America, the earliest Spanish invaders are said to have found coconuts growing along the western coast of Panama. They subsequently introduced it to Puerto Rico.

The Portuguese explorer Vasco da Gama, who was the first European to reach India by sea and link Europe and Asia by an ocean route, located coconuts on an island off Mozambique in the 15th century. Then Portuguese explorers introduced coconuts to Brazil in the 16th century. However, it wasn't until the 19th century that cultivation spread throughout Florida.

Today, the main growing and exporting countries of coconuts are Brazil, the Caribbean, India, Indonesia, Malaysia, Mexico, Papua New Guinea, the Philippines, Sri Lanka, and East and West Africa.

Coconut Geography

Coconut palms thrive along seascapes. Coconut palms are usually tall and prefer light, salty, and sandy conditions with airy soil, achieved by the ebb and tide of the neighboring seawater. The tree has shallow, widely spread roots that allow the coconut palms to gently sway, while the huge leaves (often 20 feet long with massive midribs for stability) also provide needed shade from the penetrating tropical sun for the coconut palms.

Harvesting and Using Coconuts

The coconut is the world's largest—and some say the most important and useful—nut. It's not just humans who think so: When not harvested

Hawaii, India, Indonesia, the Philippines, and parts of South America produce more than 20 billion coconuts each year.

by humans, coconuts may be picked by local monkeys right off of the palm trees.

In modern coconut plantation where dwarf cultivars of coconuts are grown, coconuts may be harvested directly from the ground with hooked knives attached to bamboo poles.

The coconut requires a sharp strike of force to split it open for its meat and water. A spike or machete is traditionally used to strike the end of the coconut and remove the husk. The coconut husk contains useful fibers known as *coir* that are used for coconut matting, among other purposes.

The "meat" or *copra,* located within the interior of the coconut, is firm and creamy white in texture and snowy white in appearance.

Also inside of the coconut is a hollowed center that is filled with a sweet, watery liquid called coconut water. Coconut water is sometimes referred to as coconut "milk," but it is really a thin liquid. If the nut is "green" or young, once it is pried open, then the refreshing coconut water is released. A sharp instrument is generally pierced into the coconut "eyes" to enable the coconut water to be poured out or for a straw to be inserted. Once mature, the dried coconut meat or copra may yield some additional coconut water.

In addition to coconut "meat" and coconut water, coconuts produce a wide array of products that include coconut "cream," coconut "milk," and coconut "oil". Coconuts provide nourishment both as a food and as a beverage, fuel for cooking, and a vessel for serving. Coconuts also produce basket materials, chemicals, medicines, textile fibers, thatching, timber, and other useful and valued products that are described in more detail in chapter 10.

A Nutritional Nut

Aside from their most notable taste and aroma, coconuts have been valued for centuries for their nutrients—particularly for their fats with energy and health-enhancing benefits. The calories contained within coconuts from fats, carbohydrates, and proteins are impressive.

One medium coconut (397 grams) contains about 1,405 calories, with:

• 133 grams of total fat (204 percent of the Daily Value [DV] based on a 2,000 daily calorie diet)

• Zero cholesterol

• 60 grams of carbohydrates (144 percent of the Daily Value)

• 36 grams of dietary fiber

• 25 grams of naturally occurring sugars

• 13 grams of protein (26 percent of the Daily Value).

What is particularly impressive about the nutrients in coconuts are the types of fats. Within 133 grams of total fat, one medium coconut contains about 118 grams of saturated fats (590 percent of the Daily Value), 1.5 grams of polyunsaturated fats and 6 grams of monounsaturated fats. While these amounts may seem high, there are good explanations about these fats and why they are considered to be so important for diet and health. A thorough explanation of dietary fats and cardiovascular disease and weight control are found in chapters 4 and 5.

Other nutrients in one medium coconut include:

• Calcium (5 percent of the Daily Value)

• Vitamin C (21 percent of the Daily Value)

• Iron (53 percent of the Daily Value)

• Vitamin B-6 (10 percent of the Daily Value)

• Magnesium (31 percent of the Daily Value)

While it is rare that a person consumes an entire medium coconut at one time, even in smaller amounts coconuts provide a proportional array of these nutrients.

What You'll Find in This Book

The *Healing Power of Coconut* celebrates the coconut, from its long and varied history and multiple, universal uses to its countless health and wellness applications and other virtues.

People have bad hair or skin days depending on where they live, their diet, and lifestyle—even their genes. Weight loss and weight maintenance, cardiovascular and brain health, and anti-aging are on-going concerns.
An array of products and procedures in today's real and virtual marketplaces promise better health, transformation, and longevity. Fine-looking skin, hair, and nails, improved defense against disease, and a youthful demeanor are on many wish lists—not to mention the satisfaction of getting these things through tasty foods and beverages.

The media extolls the next-best manufactured personal care products, and the public eagerly tries one solution after another. But

Mother Nature has packaged an array of impressive beauty and health-enhancing benefits into natural foods and beverages—the coconut being one of her finest examples.

More than that, the coconut is incredibly versatile—it supplies materials for countless uses, from simple brushes to strong ropes, furniture and car polish, and even serving bowls. How many delicious tasting foods or beverages can boast all of these attributes?

In this book you'll learn about many more fascinating ways that coconuts come to the rescue everyday for home, work, and health. You'll soon want to savor its goodness, sample its many benefits, and discover more its uses on your own.

Here's a taste of what's to come:

Chapter 2: Coconut Basics

Is the coconut is a fruit, nut, seed or all of these classifications? The unique categorization of coconuts will be featured in this chapter. You'll learn that coconuts have been staples in the diets of many cultures for thousands of years, why they were so popular, and how they are used throughout the world today.

This chapter introduces some of the many different people from around the globe who consider the coconut as a staple in their diet, including the Veddas of Sri Lanka and native Hawaiians. Could their lower incidences of heart disease be related to their coconut consumption?

The different forms of coconut, including coconut meat, milk, oil and water are featured, along with the processes that are involved in each of these products. The differences in types of coconut oil, including cold-pressed, expeller-pressed, refined, unrefined, virgin and extra-virgin are also highlighted, as well as whether or not any of these types of coconut oil have advantages over the others.

Chapter 3: How Do Coconuts Help Health?

We're taught that saturated fats are bad, which might make us want to steer clear of the coconut. But this chapter describes how the saturated fats in coconuts are different than some other saturated fats. Some dietary fats are essential to the human body and diet—contrary to the past low-fat diet craze.

Dietary fats are essential for normal physiological activities such as brain function, energy production, and a healthy immune system, but eating the right types of dietary fats and the total amount of fat in one's diet matter.

The spelling *cocoanut* is an archaic form of the word coconut. The more modernized word coconut is derived from the 15th century Portuguese and Spanish word *coco* that was used by seamen and translates to goblin, head, monkey or skull. This is because the markings on the stem end of coconuts are said to resemble facial features. The embryo of a coconut is buried

within one of the eyes of the face of the stem end. It grows though it when it sprouts!

Carl Linnaeus, the Swedish botanist physician and zoologist who formalized the modern system of naming organisms called binomial nomenclature, dubbed the coconut tree *cocos* in the 18th century. Linnaeus was also thought to have considered the word *coccus* or berry in Latin.

You could even call the coconut the "coker-nut", which is an old variation of the word coconut that was used commercially in the Port of London.

The medium-chain triglycerides (MCTs) that are found in coconuts are considered to be healthy fats. In this chapter, you'll learn why they're thought to be more beneficial than some other types of fats.

The digestive process of different kinds of fats will be simplified in this chapter to help illustrate why the medium chain triglycerides that are found in coconuts and other foods such as some butters, cheese, and yogurts may have advantages over other types of dietary fats.

Chapter 4: I Heart Coconut

This chapter focuses on examples that demonstrate the cardiovascular benefits of coconuts. Some research has shown that the dietary fats that are found in coconuts do not contribute to cardiovascular disease; rather, they may protect the heart and prevent cardiovascular disease. Once again, the medium-chain triglycerides in coconuts are central to this discussion.

Coconuts are thought to increase the levels of high-density lipoproteins (HDLs or "good" cholesterol) and lower the levels of low-density lipoproteins (LDLs or "bad" cholesterol) in the human body and they may also help

to lower blood pressure. All three measures are considered to be heart healthy. The roles that coconuts play in reaping these heart-healthy benefits will be discussed—especially in comparison to populations where coconut consumption is prominent and heart disease, in particular, is lower than in the US.

Chapter 5: Fat to Fight Fat?

Even with their higher-fat content, coconuts have been shown to aid weight loss. This chapter details the various ways that coconuts may help to fight fatness that is rapidly becoming a universal epidemic. For example, the medium-chain triglycerides that are found in coconut oil may actually help to burn stored fat and boost metabolism. Using coconut oil in cooking instead of other fats and oils may actually result in a *thermogenic* effect, in that it may help to increase energy and accelerate metabolism.

Coconut has been shown to help breakdown excess abdominal fat that is an established risk factor for cardiovascular disease and diabetes. Additionally, the consumption of coconuts may lead to satiety or a feeling of fullness and to reduced appetite. In turn, this may result in fewer calories consumed with greater enjoyment.

While the fats in coconut may help with weight loss and management, it is important to recognize that these fats contain about the same number of calories per gram (9 calories/gram) as any other fat or oil, so they should still be consumed in moderation. You'll hear about smart ways to incorporate coconuts and their healthy fats into diets without being too excessive.

This chapter also examines some of the properties of coconut water. Unlike coconut oil, coconut water is fat-free. It is also lower in calories and higher in many nutrients such as magnesium, potassium, and vitamin C. Coconut water can be used for hydration, especially as a substitute for sugary and caloric sports drinks. Like other forms of coconut, tasty

coconut water is also reported to have cardiovascular protective benefits.

Chapter 6: Use Your Brain

Some past and evolving research about coconuts involves the possible links between coconut oil and decreased risks of dementia and epilepsy. Much of the research surrounds the *ketogenic* diet, which is higher in fat and lower in carbohydrates than a typical US diet. Ketogenic diets tend to encourage the human body to burn fat for energy instead of carbohydrates, the body's preferred fuel.

This chapter describes the ketogenic diet in detail, how coconuts may conform with ketogenic diets, and why ketogenic diets may be beneficial for certain disorders affecting the brain.

For example, the effectiveness of ketogenic diets in reducing the seizures of children with epilepsy has been demonstrated. This promising discovery has prompted scientists to theorize that coconut oil with its medium-chain triglycerides may be useful for people with Alzheimer's disease and other forms of dementia.

This chapter will delve into this provocative research and pose some food for thought. It will also describe ways that coconuts may nourish the aging brain and possibly provide protection to it in order to help protect your mind and memory.

Chapter 7:
Things That Go Bump

This chapter explores the many various ways that coconut can be used for host of maladies, including minor bumps and bruises. The antimicrobial properties in coconuts will be described and how they may be beneficial for a multitude of minor ailments.

For instance, coconut oil may be used to sooth bee stings, bug bites, and simple scrapes and scratches. It can be applied as an insect repellant and has been used to prevent or treat lice infestation.

When ingested, the antibacterial and antiviral properties of coconuts may protect against common colds and strengthen the immune system. The many practical and economical uses of coconuts and solutions for common ailments are featured in this chapter—some ancient, others more modern.

Chapter 8:
Coconut the Beautiful

Coconut oil, like some other tropical oils, has been used for various beauty rituals for centuries. This chapter explains how the unique properties of coconut oil make it very versatile and useful for a myriad of beauty and hygienic practices.

Coconut oil helps to hydrate the skin, may delay aging skin with its supply of antioxidants, has antibacterial and antifungal properties, and conveys a pleasant fragrance.

Due to its versatility, coconuts can be used as a body moisturizer, hair conditioner, lip balm, makeup remover, manicure aid, moisturizer, shave lotion, and many more applications. Coconut oil can also be used for acne since its antibacterial properties are reported to help clear up the skin without clogging the pores. Coconut oil has a SPF of about 4, so it may be used as a mild, natural sunscreen.

Chapter 9: Oil-Pulling

One or the more unusual uses of coconuts is the ritual of oil pulling, which has been practiced for thousands of years in some parts of the world and has recently become more popularized in Western countries.

Practitioners of oil pulling swish coconut oil in their mouths for several minutes (sometimes as long as 20 minutes). This practice is said to improve gum health, kill bacteria, prevent cavities, and strengthen teeth.

However, the American Dental Association does caution against this oil-pulling because it has not been researched in depth and many who have attempted it say they have not noticed improvements in their overall mouth health. Nevertheless, this practice of oil-pulling coconut oil will be explored in this chapter, along with the pros and cons, to help you to formulate your own opinion.

Chapter 10:
A Natural Alternative

While the coconut contributes impressive and health benefits, there are many other unexpected ways that versatile coconuts can be used in daily life. It can be used as a natural product in cleaning and maintaining household items.

Chapter 11:
Protecting Your Pet

Don't keep the health benefits of coconut to yourself—share them with your furry friends!

Chapter 12:
Putting It All Together

We'll leave you with some last tips for coconut use, as well as tips for buying, storing, toasting, and cracking coconuts. The coconut is Mother Nature's one-stop beauty counter, hardware store, pantry, and pharmacy all packaged into one fruit, nut, and seed. Incredible coconuts help to add flavor, texture, and nourishment to foods and beverages, beautify and nourish the hair and skin, prevent and treat common health problems, supercharge the metabolism, take care of your car and home, and more.

To whet your appetite for what's to come, enjoy this tasty recipe for Date-Nut Granola. It combines melted coconut oil with old-fashioned oats, barley flakes, almonds, honey, vanilla, and dates for wholesome goodness. For a vegan version, the honey can be replaced with agave nectar or maple syrup. And for a "coconutty" touch, dried coconut "meat" can be added to the mixture before baking. Eat and enjoy!

Date-Nut Granola

⅓ cup melted coconut oil

2 cups old-fashioned oats

2 cups barley flakes

1 cup sliced almonds

⅓ cup honey

1 teaspoon vanilla

1 cup chopped dates

1. Preheat oven to 350°F. Grease 13×9-inch baking pan.

2. Combine oats, barley flakes and almonds in large bowl. Combine oil, honey and vanilla in small bowl; mix well. Pour honey mixture over oat mixture; stir until blended. Spread in prepared pan.

3. Bake about 25 minutes or until toasted, stirring frequently after first 10 minutes. Stir in dates while mixture is still hot. Cool completely; store in airtight container.

Makes 6 cups

Coconut Basics

What is basic about the coconut? Hardly anything at all! Coconuts are very simple, yet very complex in character. Understanding the inner workings of coconuts is key to appreciating their impressive characteristics and benefits.

Unique Classification

Coconuts are uniquely classified as a seed, fruit, and nut. This is because a coconut is the stone or seed of a *drupe* or fleshy fruit (the seed-bearing structure of a flowering plant) that is capable of reproducing. The word "drupe" is derived from the Latin word *drūpa* or *druppa*, which translates to overripe olive.

The fruit grows on the *Cocos nucifera*, tree-like palms that are part of the Arecaceae palm family and the only species of the Cocos genus. These palms are more closely related to grasses than they are to nut trees. However, the coconut is also considered a nut, which is a fruit that is composed of a hard, tough shell that encapsulates an edible kernel.

Structure

Coconuts are encircled by a smooth, deep tan hard outer covering that encloses the husk and a thick and fibrous layer of fruit and milk. The outside husk of a coconut is called the *exocarp,* or outer layer. The exocarp is smooth and very strong. It is green to reddish brown in color, and grays as a coconut matures. In some varieties of coconuts, the exocarp is ivory in color. The husk has three indented "eyes" at one end of the coconut.

The husk is lined with a thin brown skin called the testa that firmly adheres to the hollow kernel that is filled with coconut water. The *mesocarp* (fleshy middle layer) is thick and filled with coarse brown fibers. Within the hairy husk is the *endocarp* (a hard, woody layer that surrounds the seed) that is filled with coconut meat and milk.

Development

Coconuts originate and develop over the course of a year. A coconut is filled with liquid after about four months and attains its full size around five months when its meat becomes jelly-like.

Immature coconuts are about five to seven months old and are filled with sweet coconut water that contains about two percent sugars. Immature coconuts also contain fragile, gelatinous, moist meat that is composed of sugars and other carbohydrates and water.

Coconuts are considered to be mature after about 11 to 12 months of growth. They may weigh about 2 to 5 pounds and contain about 15 percent water, with one-quarter of their total weight composed of creamy, gelatinous, textured coconut meat. As coconuts continue to age, the meat becomes more solid and lightly fibrous.

As the coconut meat develops its fatty, firm, and white characteristics, the coconut liquid becomes less plentiful than within immature coconuts. At this stage of development, mature coconut meat is comprised of about 45 percent water, 35 percent fat, 10 percent carbohydrates, and 5 percent protein. The liquid provides a sweet and refreshing drink—often called coconut juice or simply coconut water.

Tall, Dwarf, and Hybrid

Coconuts differ in the regions where they grow throughout the world, which also determines their size, shape, and edible and usable qualities.

In general, coconuts can be classified as tall, dwarf, or hybrid. **Tall coconut palm trees** include the Jamaican Tall, Panamanian Tall, West African Tall, and the Mancapuno coconuts from the Philippines. Tall coconut palms are also found in India, Indonesia, Malaysia, New Guinea, Sri Lanka, and Tahiti.

Tall coconut palm trees are generally long-lived palm trees: to an age of about 80 to 90 years. They attain an average height of about 49 to 59 feet (15 to 18 meters) in height. Tall coconut palm trees thrive well under different soil conditions and grow well at an altitude of about 3,000 feet above sea level. They begin to bear fruit about 8 to 10 years after planting and are fairly resistant to diseases and pests.

The coconuts from tall coconut palm trees are medium-to-large in size and they vary from spheroid to linear-oblong in shape, in colors that range from green, yellow, and orange to brown. About 6,000 of these coconuts yield about a ton of copra.

Dwarf coconut palm trees include the *Cocos Niño* of the Philippines and the Dwarf Malay Golden and Dwarf Malay Green of the Caribbean. Dwarf coconut palm trees can also be found in Brazil, Fiji, India, Malaysia, Sri Lanka, and Thailand.

In contrast to tall coconut pam trees, dwarf coconut palm trees are smaller in stature (16 to 23 feet or 5 to 7 meters) and bear fruit earlier than tall coconut palm trees. On the average, dwarf coconut palm trees flower as early as three years after planting and bear their fruit in the ninth year of their average life span of 40 to 50 years. They produce green, orange, and yellow nuts that are small in size, ovoid or round in shape, and susceptible to drought. The coconuts from dwarf coconut palm trees weigh about 3 ounces and have about 65 per cent coconut oil content.

Ra Ramon coconuts from the Philippines bear the largest known coconuts. King Coconuts from Sri Lanka are known for their liquid with high sugar content. Maldivian Coconuts from the Maldives may contain the smallest of fruits, as they are no larger than eggs.

Hybrid coconut palm trees are the result of a cross between two structurally different forms of coconut. They are generally produced by two methods: with tall coconut palm trees as the female parent and dwarf coconut palm trees as the male parent (Tall x Dwarf) or dwarf coconut palm trees as the female parent and tall coconut palm trees as the male parent (Dwarf x Tall).

Hybrid coconut palm trees tend to flower early and have increased yield and better quality of copra and coconut oil when compared to their parental varieties. They also tend to grow well with the proper nutrient management and irrigation.

Worldwide Coconut Development

Humans have been transporting and cultivating coconuts around the world for ages. Coconuts were probably first cultivated in the Pacific and Indian Ocean basins, according to DNA analysis of coconuts that were collected around the world. In the Pacific Ocean basin, coconuts were likely first cultivated in Southeast Asian Islands, including Indonesia, Malaysia, and the Philippines, and perhaps on the Asian mainland. In the Indian Ocean basin, the southern border of India, including Sri Lanka, the Maldives, and the Laccadives, were likely the centers of coconut cultivation.

Coconuts from the western Indian Ocean, specifically Madagascar and the Comoros Islands, are an exception to the theories about Pacific Ocean and Indian Ocean basin cultivation. These coconuts are a genetic mixture of the Indian Ocean basin and Pacific basin coconuts and were probably first introduced and cultivated during pre-Columbian times by ancient Austronesians (from continental Asia, Madagascar, Maritime Southeast Asia, and the Islands of the Pacific Ocean). The Austronesians then established trade routes that connected and transported Southeast Asia to Madagascar and coastal east Africa. Their descendants are still living in Madagascar today. It has been reported that some coconut trees on Madagascar are genetic mixtures of the Pacific and Indian varieties.

Western Coconut Expansion

During the Spanish Colonial Era (about 1521 to 1898), the Spanish brought coconuts from the Pacific Ocean basin (especially from the Philippines) to the Pacific coast of Mexico that was governed for a period of time on behalf of the King of Spain. Some coconuts also appear to have been transported there during pre-Columbian times by the ancient Austronesians who traveled east rather than west. In Mexico today, the genetic diversity of coconut palms between ecotypes of different origins has evolved from these early introductions to its shores.

The Indian Ocean basin coconuts were transported to the New World by European explorers probably during the Age of Exploration from about the end of the 15th century to the 18th century. For example, Portuguese explorers transported coconuts from the Indian Ocean basin to the West Coast of Africa where that were later carried to the Caribbean and coastal Brazil.

This is why you may find Pacific-type coconuts on the Pacific coast of Central America and Indian-type coconuts on the Atlantic coast. The coconuts that are found in Florida today are largely the Indian Ocean basin type, in the *niu kafa* form, although several cultivars of coconut palms are grown. Niu kafa coconuts are ancestral, naturally evolved, wild coconuts that are scattered by floating. They are angular and elongated and up to six-inches in diameter, with a small egg-shaped nut that is encased by a thick husk. Niu kafa coconuts are desirable for their endosperm (meat and milk).

Dietary Staple

Coconuts have been a staple food and beverage in the diets of many cultures for thousands of years, in Polynesia, Hawaii, and Sri Lanka.

Polynesians

The Pukapuka and Tokelau of Polynesia who live on atolls near the equator consume diets that are high in saturated fat, but low in dietary cholesterol and sucrose. Coconut is their main source of calories. Vascular disease is uncommon among these Polynesians and there is little evidence of their high saturated fat intake having harmful effects.

There are two distinctively different forms of coconuts that are consumed in Polynesia: the *niu kafa* and *niu vai*, Samoan names for these Polynesian varieties.

In the late 1700s, Captain William Bligh of the British Royal Navy allegedly pitched coconuts overboard while sailing in the South Pacific. Reportedly, the historic event of the "Mutiny of the Bounty" in April 28, 1789 was prompted by Captain Bligh's harsh punishment of the mutineers for the theft of coconuts from the ship's store.

The niu kafa coconuts of Polynesia (as the coconuts that made their way to Florida) are triangular and oblong with large fibrous husks. This is in comparison to the niu vai coconuts that are rounded and brightly colored green, red, or yellow when unripe, with plenty of sweet coconut water inside.

Hawaiians

The first Hawaiian Island settlers who arrived from the Marquesas Islands around 300 to 400 AD are thought to have been of Polynesian descent. They likely brought *Niu*, the coconut that was elevated from just an ordinary food to a sacred tree in the Hawaiian Islands.

Niu is depicted in mythical art and verbal lore as a magical tree that is an image of *Ku*, the Hawaiian ancestor and the link to their heritage and life itself. Niu was valued cargo since it was considered to be the most useful plant of the tropics. There are stories of Hawaiian islanders who survived months of drought by consuming coconut water. Ancient Hawaiians were said to be strong and sturdy from their native diet, which was considered one of the best in the world for the time.

Sri Lankans

The Veddas or "Forest People" are indigenous people of Sri Lanka. The majority of Sri Lankans are of the Sinhalese race that migrated from India around two thousand years ago.

Coconut palms were very important to the Veddas for their steady source of food and drink, as well as materials that were used for building fires, eating utensils, rope, and tools.

The majority of dietary fat in the traditional Vedda diet was derived from coconuts and wild game that are both high in saturated fats. In the 1980s the Veddas were studied to determine how their high-fat diet affected their health. Their rate of cardiovascular disease was very low. Heart disease and stroke were also virtually non-existent in Kitava, Papua New Guinea, where coconuts, fish, fruit, and tubers are the main dietary staples.

While these indigenous populations survived and thrived on coconut meat and coconut water, it is important to note that their lifestyles were very different from typical North American lifestyles today, with much more activity and a less-processed diet without many of the stresses of modern society. While it is easy to make correlations between coconut consumption and decreased or absent diseases of affluence (such as cardiovascular disease, diabetes ,or hypertension), one needs to keep the isolation and location of population groups such as the Veddas in mind. Still, the low cardiovascular disease rate despite the high saturated fat consumption of the Veddas is an impressive trait worth studying.

Coconut Forms and Processes

The majority of people around the world do not cultivate their own coconuts today; rather, they purchase them whole, cracked, or dried, or as coconut oil or coconut water. Here are some of the products on the market today.

Cocolait is commercially produced coconut milk that has been nutritionally configured to resemble cow's milk.

Coconut cream is a coconut-flavored liquid that contains less water than coconut milk, which results in a more concentrated consistency and flavor. Coconut cream may also be solid and require reconstitution with warm to hot water.

Coconut gelatin (*nato de coco*) is a moist, translucent mass of cellulose or linked sugars. It is produced by a vinegar bacterium (*Acetobacter xylinum*) on the surface of coconut water that ferments.

Coconut gelatin has a crunchy texture and little flavor. Once its vinegary flavor is removed, flavor is then added and it is packed in sugar syrup to be consumed as a sweet. Coconut gelatin produced in this manner is popular in the Philippines. It is often not exported due to its unusual consistency.

Coconut ice is usually an English confection that is prepared with grated *desiccated* (dried, grated, unsweetened) coconut, condensed milk, and sugar. The mixture forms a solid, soft candy with a chewy, slightly grainy, and soft texture. In the U.S., chocolate is sometimes added to coconut ice.

Coconut meat (*or copra*) is the edible, white "meat" of coconuts that can be consumed raw or is often shredded. Coconut meat is high in fiber, calories, and fat, mostly from saturated fats. Coconut oil is extracted from the coconut meat.

Coconut milk is a sweet, coconut-flavored liquid that is produced by pouring boiling water over shredded coconut, then cooling and straining the mixture. Coconut milk of normal thickness is produced by using twice-as-much water by volume as the amount of grated coconut. A thicker coconut milk can be made with half-as-much water. The coconut pulp can be reused in the process for culinary applications. It should be covered and refrigerated.

Coconut milk is popular in Southern Indian and Southeastern Asia cuisines. Since it is an emulsion (its fat droplets are dispersed within the coconut water), coconut milk is a handy ingredient for thickening. Coconut milk contains less protein and more fat than cow's milk, but a lower-fat variety of coconut milk is available. If the fat rises to the surface of coconut milk, then it can be removed and used as coconut oil.

Coconut oil is pressed from copra, the dried meat of coconuts, but it can also be made with fresh coconuts. Coconut oil contains natural lecithin, an emulsifier and lubricant. Lecithin is an excellent cooking oil for commercial frying because it prevents spattering and provides even frying.

Coconut oil contains a higher proportion of saturated fatty acids than some polyunsaturated oils as canola, which makes it more resistant to rancidity (the deterioration of a fat or oil that leads to unpleasant odor or flavor). Coconut oil is also used as an ingredient in some candies, cookies, and pies, as well as cosmetics, margarines, and soaps.

Coconut palm heart is a vegetable that is harvested from the growing buds and inner cores of certain palm trees that include the coconut palm tree (*Cocos nucifera*). Palm hearts may also be harvested from the Açaí, Palmito Juçara, Pejibaye, Pupunha, and Sabal palm trees.

Coconut pearls are sometimes discovered inside coconuts and may be the result of arrested germination. For this reason, coconut pearls are said to have magical and medicinal powers. Their sizes range from the equivalent of an oyster pearl to a cherry. Coconuts pearls are white or blue in color and are filled with calcium carbonate, which is also found in calcium supplements.

Coconut roots are composed of a fibrous root system that is often ground to produce tea for drinking and treating minor ailments, such as skin conditions.

Coconut water is the liquid that is contained within the shell of fresh coconuts. It is sometimes clear and sometimes cloudy, depending upon its nutrient content, with a slightly nutty and sweet taste. Coconut water was a popular drink of the ancients and still is popular today for its reported medicinal value.

Coconut shells, wood, and leaves are often used in furniture making, hut walls and roofs, and tools and flooring materials, most often in areas where coconuts are grown.

Young (baby) coconuts (*Coquitos* in Chilean) are about the size of acorns and are generally sold without husks. They are often harvested early and may still have their brown hairy husks.

White coconuts are young coconuts that have the brown hairy husks removed. This process exposes their hard inner white shell.

Whole coconuts are the stones of coconut fruit that have their husks removed. This process decreases the weight of coconuts and eases shipping and handling.

Thai Veggie Curry

2	tablespoons coconut oil
1	onion, quartered and thinly sliced
1	tablespoon Thai red curry paste (or to taste)
1	can (about 13 ounces) unsweetened coconut milk
2	red or yellow bell peppers, cut into strips
1½	cups cauliflower and broccoli florets
1	cup pea pods
1	package (about 14 ounces) tofu, pressed* and cubed
	Salt and pepper
¼	cup slivered fresh basil
	Hot cooked jasmine rice

*To press tofu, cut in half horizontally . Place tofu between layers of paper towels. Place flat, heavy object on top for 10 to 30 minutes.

1. Heat oil in wok or large skillet over medium-high heat. Add onion; cook and stir 2 minutes or until softened. Add curry paste; cook and stir to coat onion. Add coconut milk; bring to a boil, stirring to dissolve curry paste.

2. Add bell peppers, cauliflower and broccoli; simmer over medium heat 4 to 5 minutes or until crisp-tender. Stir in snow peas; simmer 2 minutes. Gently stir in tofu; cook until heated through.

3. Season with salt and pepper. Sprinkle with basil; serve with rice.

Makes 4 to 6 servings

Tip: Make sure to buy unsweetened coconut milk, which is usually sold in the Asian section of the supermarket. Other coconut products cannot be substituted.

Thai Vegetable Curry combines coconut oil and coconut milk with onions, bell peppers, cauliflower, pea pods and tofu for a mouth-watering mixture to serve over rice.

Commercially Available Coconut

Dessicated coconut is produced from the white section of the coconut kernel after the thin brown layer of skin is removed. It is generally sterilized, mixed with water into a moist pulp, and sieved for different "grades"—the finest grade referred to as "macaroon." Fine grade desiccated coconut is smaller in particle size than medium grade or coconut shreds. Desiccated coconut is typically then dried, flaked, or grated. It is unsweetened and has about three percent moisture content.

Dried coconut meat (or copra) or dried coconut kernel can be pressed for its oil for use in cooking and soap making.

Fresh coconut meat is available all year; however its peak season is considered to be October through December. Fresh coconuts are best when they are heavy for their size and sound full of liquid when shook. Fresh coconut "eyes" should not be damp as coconut water might be leaking and lead to spoilage.

Depending upon their degree of ripeness, fresh coconuts may last about 6 months if left untouched at room temperature. Once the thin juice is removed through the eyes, then the meat can be grated or chopped. Freshly grated coconut should be tightly covered and refrigerated. Then it may last up to four days and be frozen up to six months.

Packaged and canned coconut is available in bags or cans, sweetened or unsweetened, flaked or shredded, and dried, moistened, or frozen. Unopened coconut in bags may last about six months. Unopened canned coconut may last up to about 18 months at room temperature. Once opened, both types of coconut must be sealed and refrigerated or frozen since its high fat content may promote rancidity.

Coconut honey is made in a similar fashion as coconut syrup: by blending and heating coconut milk and invert sugar until the mixture is a golden syrup. Golden honey contains a little of the coconut's brown rind and is cooked longer.

Coconut jaggery is the strained, unfermented coconut sap that is boiled, crystallized, and transferred into molds. Semisolid coconut jaggery then solidifies into a crystallized hard substance that is used as a sweetening agent.

Coconut palm sugar is the crystallized form of coconut palm syrup or jaggery. It has a low Glycemic Index value. (Carbohydrates with a low GI value are more slowly digested, absorbed, and metabolized by the human body, which results in a slower rise in blood glucose and insulin levels.) Coconut palm sugar is popular in Indonesia. In the US, coconut palm sugar may be mixed with cane sugar.

Coconut syrup is made by blending and heating coconut milk and invert sugar (a mixture of the two simple sugars glucose and fructose). This process yields "golden syrup" that is similar to pure invert sugar. It is less prone to crystallization, moist, sweet, and valued by bakers.

Coconut toddy is an alcoholic beverage that is made by tapping the coconut tree by cutting off the tips of the flowing stems. Once fermented, this beverage can be consumed raw or distilled to produce *arak* (a Levantine alcoholic spirit that is anise-flavored, clear, colorless, and unsweetened). It can also be used as a source of yeast in bread making or it can be fermented further into vinegar.

Types and Advantages of Coconut Oil

Coconut oil is generally liquid at room temperature, though this characteristic may change depending upon its country of origin. However, it solidifies at temperatures below that, so refrigerated or frozen coconut oil will look quite dense.

After processing, coconut oil is almost tasteless, so it is commonly used in baked goods, confections, cooking oils, and margarines for its great versatility.

There are several types of coconut oil, mostly distinguished by the types or lack of processing.

Unrefined coconut oil, also called "pure" or "virgin" coconut oil, is made from fresh coconut meat instead of dried. The coconut oil is extracted by either a quick-dry method or through a wet-milling process.

Quick drying dries the coconut meat rapidly; then the coconut oil is pressed out mechanically. *Wet milling* first processes the coconut meat into coconut milk. Then the coconut milk is separated from the coconut oil by boiling, centrifuging, fermenting, straining, or by the use of enzymes.

Because both of these extraction methods are quick, the coconut oil does not require additives or bleaching. Both processes also retain more flavor since they do not expose the coconut oil to high temperatures.

Refined coconut oil is made from dried coconut meat, or copra. (Some copra-based refined coconut oils are referred to as "RBD oils" since they are **r**efined, **b**leached and **d**eodorized). The coconut meat is bleached (generally not by a chemical process, but by filtration) and treated to reduce any bacteria. However, the drying process itself may produce contaminants.

A high heat process is then used to extract the coconut flavor and aroma. Sometimes chemicals are used to extract as much oil as possible. Sodium hydroxide may be added to increase shelf life. Refined coconut oil is sometimes partially hydrogenated, but this process may produce trans fats, which are disallowed in United States manufacture by the U.S. Food and Drug Administration (USFDA).

Virgin coconut oil is derived from the expeller pressing of coconut oil from dried (desiccated) coconut. It is not distinguished by an industry standard, much like in the olive oil industry; however, it is considered to be unrefined.

Extra-virgin coconut oil, similar to virgin coconut oil, bears little distinction to extra-virgin olive oil or any oil with an "extra-virgin" designation. It implies that this type of coconut oil has the highest quality and retains the original chemical composition and nutritive values of coconuts. Unlike olive oil there is no industry standard definition.

Cold-pressed coconut oil is produced at low temperature from fresh, dried coconut flakes. It has a stronger coconut flavor than expeller-pressed coconut oil and may contain tiny traces of soluble components that are extracted from the dried coconut meat. Cold-pressed coconut oil is considered as "raw" coconut oil. Since it is not exposed to high heat, many of its nutrients may be retained so it may be preferable to other choices.

Expeller-pressed coconut oil is produced through a mechanical extraction process that does not rely upon solvent extracts or other chemical processes. Expeller-pressed coconut oil has less of a coconut taste than cold-pressed coconut oil, but it has a higher smoke point that makes it desirable for cooking.

Centrifuge extracted coconut oil is made from freshly pressed coconut milk that is chilled and separated by centrifugal force. Like cold-pressed coconut oil, centrifuge-extracted coconut oil is considered as a raw coconut oil because it retains mostly all of its nutrients during processing. It has a light coconut flavor and may be quite expensive, likely due to its nutrient retention and subtle taste and aroma.

Organic coconut oil should be produced under organic standards, unrefined, and pressed at low heat to retain its antioxidants and *phenols*, biologically active compounds. Select unhydrogenated organic coconut oil without trans fats (which must appear on the nutrition label). Refrigerate after opening.

Some refined coconut oils, especially those that are used in chocolate production and commercial baking, may be partially hydrogenated.

Coconut Cost

Coconuts are relatively inexpensive in cost—that is, if one lives in India, Indonesia, Mexico, or Thailand. Because coconuts have become so popular, prices have soared and are continuing their upward trend. In particular, the sale of coconut water is a rising industry.

The coconut plantations in the Caribbean are experiencing a shortage and those in the Philippines have faced natural disasters, raising prices. Still, coconuts are relatively economical in their natural state.

In Hawaii, a coconut may cost about $2.00, but once it is opened and processed, then the price may escalate (one pound of organic coconut shreds could cost as much as $10.00 a bag). A metal coconut opener may be pricy, but a stake of some kind should be able to poke open a coconut through one of its "eyes".

Coconut milk and coconut water may range in price depending upon the size and type of packing and manufacturer. Pricy coconut water is fashionable, but the cost per nutrient may not make sense.

Bottom line: Coconuts may require some "elbow grease" to pry open; still, they are economical for all of their benefits.

Availability

If one lives in the southeast or southwest and along the coastlines, then coconut palms may be familiar sights. Coconuts may be so abundant that they drop off their branches on to the ground to be scooped up for cracking, munching fresh coconut meat, or sipping refreshing coconut water.

Around the world coconuts, coconut milk, coconut water and other forms of coconuts may be instantly purchased and promptly delivered. Mass food markets now sell coconuts and coconut products to meet consumer demand for coconut's beauty, culinary, health, and home usages. Due to their popularity, the accessibility makes coconuts different than some other hard-to-purchase foods or beverages. It's easy to access the benefits of coconuts!

How Do Coconuts Help Health?

In this chapter, we'll look at five notable features of the incredible coconut that point to its healing properties.

1. Saturated fats

The word is that fat is bad for us, and saturated fat especially, so how are the saturated fats in coconut different than other saturated fats in foods and beverages? This chapter discusses how, contrary to what the diet industry has the public believing, fat is needed in the daily diets. This nutrient is essential for processes such as brain function, energy production, and immune protection. Still, it is vital to consume the right kinds of fats and in the right amounts.

The "medium-chain triglycerides" (MCTs) that are found in coconuts (and discussed in many chapters throughout this book—particularly in chapters 4, 5, and 6) are considered to be more beneficial than some other kinds of fats and for good reason. For instance,

medium-chain triglycerides are more easily digested and immediately converted to energy, whereas "long-chain triglycerides" (LCTs), which make up the majority of the fat in our diets, are carried by the bloodstream and are not necessarily burned for energy. This chapter will distinguish among these types of fats and more to illustrate why the coconut is a cut above other foods of its kind.

Chemically speaking, saturated fats are fat molecules that are saturated with hydrogen molecules. Practically speaking, saturated fats are fats that are filled to capacity and are difficult for the body to disengage.

Saturated fats have been on the nutrition and health radar for years due to their relationship to cardiovascular disease. The reason why saturated fats are discouraged is that they tend to raise the level of cholesterol in the blood-stream, which in turn may increase a person's risk of cardiovascular disease and stroke. Conversely, replacing foods and beverages that are higher in saturated fats with those that are lower in saturated fats may lower serum (blood) cholesterol, improve lipid profiles in the blood, and conceivably even reduce the risks of cardiovascular disease and stroke. The *lipid profile* is a panel of blood tests that provides a screening tool for blood lipids that include cholesterol and triglycerides.

Polyunsaturated fats are fat molecules that have openings in their structures without hydrogen molecules. They tend to be lighter fats and are thought to be health enhancing. Polyunsaturated fats are sometimes made into saturated fats through the process of *hydrogenation,* as discussed in Chapter 4. Hydrogenation adds more hydrogen to fat molecules to make them more stable.

Consider canola oil. Through hydrogenation, canola oil could become hydrogenated into canola oil-based margarine, transformed from tub to stick. In the process, artificial trans fats are formed, which have been deemed un-safe by the U.S. Department of Agriculture.

Currently the American Heart Association (AHA) offers recommendations that Americans should aim for a dietary pattern that contains five to six percent of calories from saturated fat. If a person consumes 2,000 calories daily (the figure that the U.S. Food and Drug Administration use to determine the Daily Values [DVs] of different nutrients), then this means that no more than about 120 calories or 13 grams of saturated fats should be consumed daily.

Also according to the American Heart Association, a daily diet pattern should emphasize fruits, vegetables, whole grains, low-fat dairy products, poultry, fish, and nuts and limit red meats and sugary foods and beverages. The AHA also suggests that foods with high monounsaturated and/or polyunsaturated fatty acids should replace foods that are higher in saturated fatty acids.

Saturated fats occur naturally in foods and beverages. The majority of saturated fats are derived from animal sources, particularly meats and dairy products. Beef fat (tallow), butter, cheese, and other dairy products that are made with two percent or whole milk, fatty beef, lard, lamb, pork, and poultry with skin are examples of animal products that contain saturated fats.

Some plant-based oils such as coconut oil, palm oil, and palm kernel oil do not contain cholesterol (a fatty substance that is also a risk factor in cardiovascular disease and stroke), but they do primarily contain saturated fats.

Coconuts, Saturated Fats, Health, and Heart Disease

What might be considered as an enigma to this discussion about the relationship between saturated fats and cardiovascular disease and stroke is the relationship of coconuts and cardiovascular and brain health that will be described more fully in later chapters.

Out of the 133 grams of total fat in one medium coconut, 118 grams or roughly 88.7 percent is from saturated fats. This is approximately 590 percent of the Daily Value that is based on a 2,000 daily calorie diet. In comparison, the amount of polyunsaturated fat is only 1.5 grams and the amount of monounsaturated fat is only 6 grams.

Also in comparison, the amount of saturated fat in butter is about 64 percent of total calories and the amount of saturated fat in beef fat is about 40 percent of total calories, or about the same amount as in lard.

What is different about the saturated fats in coconut oil is that these fats tend to increase high-density lipoprotein cholesterol (or HDL–the "good" cholesterol). This is based on short-term studies that examined the affects of coconut oil on serum cholesterol levels. As of last year, the exact mechanisms by which coconut oil affects cardiovascular disease were not confirmed.

The saturated fat in coconut oil is mostly comprised of medium-chain triglycerides (MCTs). These medium-chain triglycerides are handled differently in the body than the longer-chain fatty acids that are found in dairy products, fatty meals, and liquid vegetable oils. This distinction is the next notable feature of coconuts.

Coconut Curry Chicken Soup

3 cups chicken broth

8 boneless skinless chicken thighs

1 cup chopped onion, divided

1 teaspoon salt, divided

4 whole cloves

1 tablespoon coconut oil

2 tablespoons curry powder

1¼ cups coconut milk

¼ cup plus 1 tablespoon chopped fresh mint, divided

3 tablespoons crystallized ginger

¼ teaspoon ground cloves

1½ cups half-and-half

3 cups cooked rice

Lime wedges (optional)

1. Bring broth to a boil in large saucepan over high heat. Add chicken, ½ cup onion, ½ teaspoon salt and whole cloves. Return to a boil. Reduce heat to low; cover and simmer 40 minutes or until tender. Remove chicken; set aside. Strain cooking liquid; reserve 1 cup.

2. Melt coconut oil in same skillet over medium-high heat. Add remaining ½ cup onion; cook and stir 4 minutes or until onion is translucent. Sprinkle curry powder over onions; cook 20 seconds or just until fragrant, stirring constantly.

3. Add coconut milk, 1 tablespoon mint, ginger, ground cloves and reserved cooking liquid to saucepan. Cover; simmer 10 minutes. Add chicken; cover and simmer 15 minutes. Stir in half-and-half and remaining ½ teaspoon salt. Shred chicken slightly, pressing down with spoon. Cook 1 minute or until heated through. Sprinkle with remaining ¼ cup mint. Spoon rice over each serving and garnish with lime wedges.

Makes 4 servings

Coconut Curry Chicken Soup uses chicken broth, skinless chicken thighs, onions, cloves, coconut oil, curry powder, coconut milk, fresh mint, crystalized ginger, cloves and half-and-half along with cooked rice and fresh lime for a mouth-watering and tempting synthesis of tastes.

2. Medium-chain Triglycerides

Triglycerides are the most common type of fat in the body. They come from food; the human body also makes triglycerides. Once the triglycerides in foods and beverages are consumed and digested, they travel through in the blood and supply energy or are stored for future use. Foods and beverages that are higher in cholesterol and saturated fats tend to elevate serum (blood) triglyceride levels. High levels of blood triglycerides are frequently seen in people with heart problems, have diabetes, or are overweight.

There are different types of triglycerides that are differentiated according to the number and types of fatty acids, whether they are saturated or unsaturated, and their degree of unsaturation. Triglycerides are designed as short, medium, or long in length.

Short-chain triglycerides: Short-chain triglycerides are triglycerides that are generally about two to five carbon atoms in length. They are primarily absorbed through the portal vein during lipid digestion, much like medium-chain triglycerides are.

Medium-chain triglycerides (MCTs): Medium-chain triglycerides are triglycerides that are generally about 6 to 12 carbon atoms in length. The fatty acids in medium-chain triglycerides are generally broken off from their triglyceride structure without the need of bile (an alkaline fluid that aids in fat digestion) from the liver. Then the MCTs are "shuttled" via the portal artery directly to the liver without the use of chylomicrons (small, lipoprotein particles) for transport. This attribute makes medium-chain triglycerides desirable for their relatively quicker source of energy compared to long-chain triglycerides with less dependency upon the liver.

Long-chain triglycerides (LCTs): Long-chain triglycerides are triglycerides that are generally about 14 to 22 carbon atoms in length. Long-chain triglycerides usually require both bile and lipases (fat-digesting enzymes) to be emulsified and broken down into individual fatty acids in the small intestine. Then these fatty acids are reassembled and carried through the blood or lymph, used by the body as needed or stored. The process is lengthier than medium-chain triglyceride digestion, absorption, and utilization and is dependent upon bile and lipases.

What makes the types of fat in coconuts different than the fats that are found in other foods and beverages is that practically all of the fat in coconuts are medium-chain triglycerides (MCTs), while the majority of fats that are consumed by humans are long-chain triglycerides (LCTs). This factor is responsible for the unique character and healthful properties of coconut oil and has many implications.

Medium-chain triglycerides are used in hospital formulas to feed very young infants, people who are critically ill, and those who may have digestive problems. This is because MCTs are easily digested, absorbed and utilized to nourish the human body. Because of their quick conversion into energy, medium-chain triglycerides are also used by athletes, for weight management, and in the treatment of *epilepsy* in children. Epilepsy is a neurological disorder that is designated by recurrent episodes of sensory disturbances. When medium-chain triglycerides are used in conjunction with a prescribed ketogenic diet, symptoms appear to decrease. Later chapters describe the keto-genic diet in more detail.

The medium-chain triglycerides that are found in coconuts are also found in human breast milk.

What makes the medium-chain triglycerides in coconuts different is that most of the fatty acids are saturated. Other than treating epilepsy, the critically ill, those with digestive disorders, and young infants, the medium-chain triglycerides in coconuts have shown effectiveness in cardio-vascular risk prevention and health promotion. These at-tributes are opposite to the effects that other saturated fats may have on the human body and health.

This leads to another feature of the coconut that makes it different in good ways: the lauric acid content.

3. Lauric Acid

Lauric acid, a component of triglycerides, is saturated fatty acid with a 12-carbon chain, so it is considered to be a medium-chain fatty acid. Lauric acid comprises about one-half of the fatty acids in coconut milk and coconut oil (49 percent of total fat). It is also found in cow's milk (2.9 percent of total fat), goat's milk (3.1 percent of total fat) and human breast milk (6.2 percent of total fat).

A fairly recent animal study demonstrated the ability of lauric acid to reduce blood pressure, heart rate, and oxidative stress in the arteries and the kidneys.

Lauric acid increases total serum cholesterol due to its favorable increase in high-density lipoprotein cholesterol (HDL or "good" cholesterol) that correlates with decreased risks of *atherosclerosis* (hardening of the arteries) and cardiovascular disease.

Both lauric acid and monolaurin also have demonstrated antimicrobial activity against some bacteria, fungi, and viruses. This is why, along with vascular disease, lauric acid may be used to treat a host of other conditions that include the avian flu, cold sores, the common cold, fever blisters, genital herpes and warts, the swine flu, and viral infections including influenza. And this is also why coconut oil with its high percentage of lauric acid is valued by some for its antibacterial, antifungal, and antiviral properties.

4. Coconut's Nutritional Value

Some foods and beverages boast that they are Mother Nature's perfect food. While no food or beverage is 100 percent perfect, the incredible coconut provides its share of nutrients in one convenient package.

First consider coconut meat, the edible white interior of coconuts.

- It is a storehouse of energy providing 283 calories per one cup of raw, shredded coconut meat.

- It provides carbohydrates with 12 tasty grams of carbohydrates per one cup.

- It is a high source of dietary fiber with 7 grams of dietary fiber per one cup.

- It has 27 grams of total fat with 24 grams of saturated fat and no cholesterol per one cup of raw, shredded coconut meat.

- It provides 3 grams of protein per one cup.

- It is low in sodium with only 16 milligrams of sodium per one cup.

Next consider coconut milk.

• It is a storehouse of energy with 552 calories per one cup of raw coconut milk.

• It provides carbohydrates with 13 grams of carbohydrates per one cup.

• It is a good source of dietary fiber with 5 grams of dietary fiber per one cup.

• It contains 57 grams of total fat with 51 grams of saturated fat and no cholesterol.

• It provides protein with 5 grams of protein per one cup.

• It is low in sodium with only 36 milligrams of sodium per one cup.

Berry Coconut Milk Smoothie

1   cup unsweetened coconut milk

2   cups berries (blueberries, raspberries and/or strawberries)

4   to 5 whole ice cubes

1   tablespoon coconut oil (optional)

Cinnamon (optional)

1. Place the first three ingredients into a blender.

2. Blend at low speed until smooth.

3. Dribble with coconut oil, if desired.

4. Blend at medium speed until well blended.

5. Top with sprinkle of cinnamon, if desired.

Makes 2 cups

Then consider coconut water.

- It is low in calories with only 46 calories per one cup of coconut water.

- It provides carbohydrates with just 9 calories of carbohydrates per one cup of coconut water.

- It provides dietary fiber with 3 grams of dietary fiber per one cup.

- It contains zero grams of total fat, saturated fat or cholesterol.

- It provides protein with 2 grams of protein per one cup.

- Note that it is is higher in sodium at 252 milligrams per one cup.

This equates to plenty of energy from the calories in fats, carbohydrates, and proteins, plus dietary fiber and relatively little sodium with plenty of essential and supportive vitamins and minerals (to be discovered throughout this book). What other foods or beverages can boast all of these nutrients in these levels that are encapsulated into just one incredible coconut?

5. Body Benefits

What other fruit, nut, or seed has so many beauty properties can be used in so many different hygiene and beauty applications? Coconut oil can be used as a body oil, body lotion, body scrub, breath freshener, cuticle oil, make-up remover and make-up brush cleanser, dandruff treatment, deep conditioner, deodorant, frizz tamer, itch reliever, leave-in conditioner, lip balm, massage oil, night cream under eye cream, shaving cream, stretch mark cream, and teeth whitener among many other usages.

A mixture of apple cider vinegar and coconut oil when combed through hair may be effective in ridding and preventing head lice. Just ask any parent of school-aged children who have been infested with head lice: they may agree that delousing the hair with a natural product such as coconut oil may be the alternative to harsh chemical treatments.

In comparison, avocadoes are technically classified as fruit since they are large berries that contain single seeds. Like coconuts, avocadoes have a host of beauty benefits. Avocadoes contain antioxidants carotenoids that include alpha- and beta-carotene, cryptoxanthin, zeaxanthin, and lutein. These antioxidants help to protect the skin from environmental damage from oxygen-free radicals that may contribute to visible signs of aging, such as fine lines or wrinkles.

Plus, avocadoes contain vitamin C—also for healthy skin. Vitamin C is needed to create elastin and collagen that helps to bind the skin and maintain the firmness and structure of skin cells.

Another antioxidant that is found in avocadoes is vitamin E that also helps to prevent free radical damage and may be protective against excessive sun exposure.

One of the biggest beauty benefits of avocadoes is their composition of monounsaturated fatty acids from their high oleic acid content. Monounsaturated fatty acids help to moisturize the epidermal layer of the skin to keep it hydrated and soft in appearance and are said to help decrease inflammation.

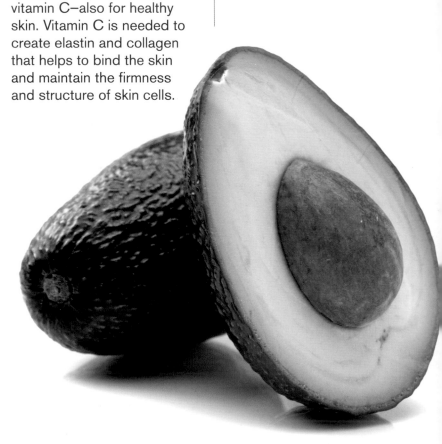

However, a virgin coconut oil-enriched diet was also shown to have a beneficial role in improving antioxidant status and preventing lipid and protein oxidation, or breakdown. Plus, the saturated fat content of coconuts has shining benefits.

The inherent saturated fats in coconuts reportedly help to strengthen the underlying tissues of the skin and remove excessive dead cells on the skin's surface, leaving it smooth and devoid of roughness and flakiness. Also, the medium-chain triglycerides act as antibacterial, antifungal, and antiviral agents to protect the skin and scalp from these menacing invaders. Lastly, coconut water with its light and refreshing coconut aroma is refreshing and hydrating for needy skin.

So while other foods and beverages may have their beauty benefits, the coconut is different: it scores threefold as a fruit, nut, and seed in the beauty world.

Not Just for Health

The benefits of coconut don't end with your health. Let's take a quick look at some of the other uses and benefits of the amazing coconut.

• One surprising use of coconuts and what makes them a standout in the plant kingdom is their use to both whiten and shine the body and the home. Who would imagine that a natural substance such as coconut oil could whiten the stains on teeth enamel *and* shine leather shoes? Or that coconut oil may moisten and shine lips *and* polish wooden floors and furniture to a warm glow? Or that coconut oil may lighten simple bruises and scrapes *and* brighten cast-iron pans?

• It is difficult to walk into a bakery or perfumery without sensing the pleasantly sweet and tropical scent of coconuts. Likewise, the taste of coconuts is so distinct that it is hard not to identify the taste of coconuts in savory or sweet foods or beverages. This can be advantageous and disadvantageous. The scent and taste of coconut are so distinct that some may either have a love or dislike for these sensations. Some subtler smelling fruits, nuts, and seeds are too difficult to detect so assertively as coconuts .

• Coconut has many culinary applications in cooking and baking. The coconut meat, milk, and water are exceptionally versatile in appetizers, breakfasts, desserts, main dishes, side dishes, smoothies, soups, and stews. Coconut meat, milk, and water add aroma, fat, moisture, taste, and texture in common and surprising ways. For example, when shredded coconut is used in baked goods the flavor is full-bodied, moist, and tropical. And when toasted coconut tops fruit or curries, browning brings out the fatty, nutty coconut taste.

I Heart Coconuts

This chapter focuses on all the ways that the coconut has been shown to protect the heart. Contrary to past thinking, research has shown that the fat in coconuts does not contribute to heart disease and on the contrary, may protect the heart and prevent heart disease.

The coconut is thought to increase levels of high-density lipoproteins (HDL or "good") cholesterol) and lower levels of low-density lipoprotein (LDL or "bad" cholesterol) and may also help to lower blood pressure.

In this chapter the roles that the coconut plays in reaping heart-healthy benefits are discussed.

Cardiovascular Disease

For more than 50 years cardiovascular disease has been one of the major causes of death in the United States. The underlying cause of cardiovascular disease is atherosclerosis, which is a condition that is characterized by plaque, or fatty deposits that are lodged within the arterial walls. Plaque interferes with blood flow to the heart and brain that may lead to a heart attack or stroke.

Diet is a modifiable cardiovascular and cerebral risk factor, meaning that when one's diet is heart-healthy then risks decrease.

Heart Disease: Terms to Know

Angina pectoris is a condition that is marked by severe chest pain and/or discomfort that often spreads to the neck and shoulders. It is frequently due to insufficient blood flow to the heart muscle that results from obstruction or spasm within the coronary arteries.

Risk factors, such as age, gender, and genetics are fixed and may either compound or reduce various cardiovascular risks. As an example, an older man with a family history of heart disease may have greater cardiovascular and cerebral risks than a younger woman without cardiovascular family incidents.

Ischemic heart disease is characterized by reduced blood supply to the heart due to narrowing of the arteries and less blood and oxygen delivered to the heart muscle. Ischemic heart disease is the most common cause of death in Western countries.

A **heart attack** is sometimes referred to as a myocardial infarction. It occurs when one or more regions of the heart have severe oxygen debt. This may be the result of blood clots that block the flow of blood through coronary arteries to the heart muscle.

The average age for a first heart attack in the U.S. is 65 years old. However, it has been estimated that four to ten percent of U.S. men aged 45 years or younger experience a heart attack and **atherosclerosis** or hardening of the arteries starts in youth.

The risk factors for heart attacks include age, autoimmune disease, diabetes, family history of heart attack, high blood cholesterol or triglyceride levels, high blood pressure, illegal drug use, lack of physical activity, obesity, preeclampsia, stress, and tobacco use.

A **stroke** occurs when the blood supply to the brain is either blocked or a blood vessel within the brain ruptures. In either instance, brain tissue may die and brain health may be compromised or this may lead to death. A stroke is considered a medical emergency and treatment is needed very quickly. It is the fifth leading cause of death in the US.

There are three main types of strokes: ischemic, hemorrhagic and mini-strokes (transient ischemic attacks). An ischemic stroke is the result of an obstruction within a blood vessel that supplies blood to the brain. A hemorrhagic stroke occurs when a weakened blood vessel ruptures. A transient ischemic attack occurs when the blood supply to the brain is briefly blocked.

In comparison to a heart attack, the risks for having a stroke of any kind doubles each decade after the age of 55 years, though strokes may occur at any age. In fact, almost one-fourth of strokes occur in the US to people under 65 years of age, especially when they have risks factors that include alcohol consumption, gender (women more than men), oral contraceptive use, post-menopausal hormone therapy, race (Asian, African-American and Hispanic in particular), tobacco use, and past heart attacks or strokes.

Coconut Consumption

Let's examine populations around the world with higher coconut consumption than in the United States and see what we can learn from these populations in terms of coconuts in history, cardiovascular disease, health, and longevity. There is a rich history of coconut consumption for nutrition, health, and well-being in countries around the world where coconuts have thrived for centuries.

Kitavans

The Kitavans who reside on the Trobriand Islands, Papua New Guinea, consume a significant amount of coconuts and reportedly exhibit excellent health. A subsistence lifestyle is still followed by Kitavan islanders. Dietary staples include coconuts, fish, fruit, and tubers. Stroke and ischemic heart disease appear to be absent in this population.

In a study that was conducted in the 1990s, when the frequencies of aphasia, exertion-related chest pain, hemiparesis, sudden imbalance, or spontaneous sudden death were assessed in Kitavan islanders, no cases that corresponded to angina pectoris, stroke, or sudden death was reported.

Pukapukas and Tokelauans

The Pukapukas and Tokelauans from the southern Pacific Ocean are also sizeable coconut consumers. Over 60 percent of their daily calorie intake is from coconuts and they reportedly have the largest saturated fat consumptions in the world with the absence of heart disease.

The diets of the atoll dwellers near the equator from both Pukapuka and Tokelau are high in saturated fats but low in dietary cholesterol and sucrose. Coconut is the main source of energy for both of these population groups.

A study from the 1980s showed that Tokelauan people acquire a higher percentage of energy (calories) from coconuts than people from Pukapuka: 63 percent compared to 34 percent, with a higher intake of saturated fat. In comparison, the serum cholesterol levels in Tokelauans were 35 to 40 milligrams higher than in the Pukapukans.

The difference in serum cholesterol level was attributed to the higher saturated fat intake of the Tokelauans due to the high lauric acid (12:0) and myristic acid (14:0) content. In both populations vascular disease is uncommon and there is no evidence of high saturated fat intake having detrimental health effects in these populations.

In order to truly understand the cardiovascular and brain benefits that the coconut consumption provides for these indigenous populations, an examination of heart-healthy diets and the heart disease process is warranted.

Heart-Healthy Diets

In the 1950s the connection between saturated fats and cardiovascular disease was widely circulated throughout the US and lower-fat diets were developed and promoted for cardiovascular disease protection.

Then, in the 1980s, the first set of U.S. Dietary Guidelines were established by the Departments of Agriculture (USDA) and Health and Human Services (HHS). These new guidelines recommended that all Americans avoid eating too much total fat, saturated fat, and cholesterol.

The U.S. Dietary Guidelines were revised every five years and Americans were advised, among other recommendations, to continue to follow lower total fat, lower saturated fat, and lower cholesterol diets.

In the 1990s, while the recommendations for dietary fats generally remained the same, the recommendation for dietary carbohydrates instructed that Americans, "Choose a diet with plenty of grain products with vegetables and fruits."

Some dietary fats in foods and beverages were replaced by carbohydrates and often by sugars. This let to recommendations to "Choose a variety of grains daily, especially whole grains; choose a variety of fruits and vegetables daily; choose beverages and foods to moderate your intake of sugars and choose a diet that is low in saturated fat and cholesterol and moderate in total fat."

These guidelines may have been misinterpreted by the U.S. public, who thought that carbohydrates could be freely consumed—as long as they were healthy whole grains. As a result, higher carbohydrate diets were popular at the close of the twentieth century.

Concurrently, fats such as butter and lard were replaced with manufactured margarines, most with trans fatty acids (which have a relationship to increased cardiovascular disease).

In conjunction with these 50 years of U.S. Dietary Guidelines, after peaking around 1968, the age-adjusted rates from cardiovascular disease were reduced in half by the year 2000. Two factors mainly contributed to this reduction: substantial decreases in elevated total cholesterol, high blood pressure, and tobacco use (major cardiovascular risk factors) and new treatments for established cardiovascular disease. These include angioplasty, bypass grafting, stents, enzyme (ACE) inhibitors, statins, and thrombolysis. Deaths from strokes also declined over this same period of time. However, the prevalence of both diabetes and obesity has alarmingly increased.

Today saturated fatty acids, such as those that are found in coconuts, are looked at differently than before for their relationship to cardiovascular disease prevention and health enhancement. An examination of differences among fatty acids helps to sort out which are healthier by today's standards and why and how coconuts fit into the total cardiovascular picture.

Lentil Vegetable Stew

Lentil Vegetable Stew combines coconut oil with cauliflower, onions, red bell pepper, tomatoes, and yellow squash with lentils for a filling, savory, and nourishing soup or entrée.

3 tablespoons coconut oil (refined)

1 large onion, coarsely chopped

1 can (28 ounces) crushed tomatoes

2 cups water

1 tablespoon curry powder

1 tablespoon cider vinegar

1½ teaspoons salt

1½ teaspoons ground cumin

1½ teaspoons ground coriander

1 teaspoon ground ginger

1¼ cups dried lentils, rinsed

2 cups cauliflower florets

1 cup chopped red bell pepper

1 cup chopped yellow squash

1. Heat oil in large saucepan over medium heat. Add onion; cook and stir 5 minutes or until softened. Stir in tomatoes, water, curry powder, vinegar, salt, cumin, coriander and ginger. Stir in lentils; bring to a boil. Reduce heat to medium-low; simmer 35 to 45 minutes or until lentils begin to soften.

2. Add cauliflower, bell pepper and squash; cook 30 to 40 minutes or until vegetables and lentils are tender.

Makes 8 servings

A Fat Primer

Cholesterol is a fatty substance that occurs in only animal foods and products. Organ meats, high-fat dairy products, and some seafood are higher in cholesterol. Cholesterol is a contributing factor in cardiovascular disease, but non-dietary factors may also raise cholesterol and increase one's predisposition to cardiovascular disease. There are primarily three types of serum cholesterol that are considered predictive of cardiovascular disease:

• **High-density lipoproteins (HDL-cholesterol)**: known as the "good cholesterol" because it proportionally carries more protein than cholesterol from the blood to the liver to be recycled or for disposal. HDL-cholesterol is affected more by a person's activity level, gender, obesity and smoking than diet.

• **Low-density lipoproteins (LDL-cholesterol)**: known as the "bad" cholesterol because it mainly carries cholesterol and is associated with increased risk of cardiovascular disease.

Dietary cholesterol, saturated fat intake, total dietary fat, trans fat, and excess calories are some of the dietary factors that are thought to increase LDL-cholesterol, in addition to the lifestyle factors of obesity, inactivity, and smoking.

• **Very-low density lipoproteins (VLDL-cholesterol)**: is also known as the "bad" cholesterol. It is produced by the liver and released into the blood to supply triglycerides (see below). High VLDL-cholesterol is associated with plaque development on artery walls that narrows and restricts blood flow. By exercising and losing weight and avoiding sugary foods and alcohol, the body's serum (blood) triglyceride level may be decreased.

Lipids are a family of fats, oils, phospholipids (such as lecithin), and sterols (such as cholesterol) that are found in plants or animals, or sometimes both. Cholesterol is only found in animals.

Sometimes lipids are inadvertently called "fats", but they really contain many more substances.

Fats are lipids that are solid at room temperature. Animal fats include bacon, butter, lard, the skin of poultry, and the fat that runs though meats. Generally speaking, the more solid the fat, the more difficult it is for the body to break down.

Hydrogenation is the process of converting unsaturated fatty acids into saturated fatty acids through a method of trans bonds. As a result, these fatty acids are very difficult for the body to break down and they may contribute to cardiovascular disease.

Partially hydrogenated means that some fatty acid bonds are "partially" hydrogenated or filled, which makes them somewhat easier to digest. Instead of risky trans bonds, partially-hydrogenated fatty acids have different linkages, or cis bonds. Some frostings, margarines, and shortenings are all foods with partially-hydrogenated products.

Phospholipids are similar in structure to triglycerides, but they also contain phosphorus. They also provide the major structural components of membranes. Lecithin is a phospholipid that naturally occurs in animals, plants (in soybeans) and eggs, among other foods. Lecithin is used as an emulsifier by the body and by the food industry.

Phospholipids in the form of lecithin are found in egg yolks, liver, peanuts, and wheat germ. They are also found in milk, soybeans, and lightly cooked meats. The human body can synthesize lecithin if there is sufficient choline in the diet from dairy foods, eggs, fish, meats, poultry, pasta, or rice.

Oils are lipids that are liquid at room temperature. They include such oils as avocado, canola, coconut, olive, peanut, and safflower. While coconut oil is semi-solid at room temperature (due to its saturated fat), it is referred to as an oil.

Essential fatty acids must be consumed by the body and are essential for its normal functioning. There are two essential fatty acids (EFAs) that cannot be synthesized by the body: *linoleic* and *alpha-linolenic*. These must be obtained by food. These two essential fatty acids are used to build omega-3 fatty acid and omega-6 fatty acid, both important in normal body functioning (see below). Salmon, herring, mackerel, hemp, flax, walnuts, almonds, dark leafy green vegetables, olive oil, whole grains, and eggs are good sources of essential fatty acids. The human body can generally produce non-essential fatty acids from other substances.

Monounsaturated fatty acids are unsaturated at one point in their fatty acid structures where they can be broken down, so they are considered to be healthier. Monounsaturated fatty acids are primarily found in canola, olive, peanut, safflower, and sesame oils, as well as in avocadoes, peanut butter, and many nuts and seeds.

Omega-3 fatty acids (Omega 3's) are essential fatty acids that are associated with heart health and disease prevention. Omega 3-fatty acids may help to decrease cholesterol and platelet clotting and inflammatory and immune reactions. They are primarily found in chia seeds, fatty fish, fish oil, flax seeds and flax oil, seafood, soybeans, spinach, and walnuts.

Omega-6 fatty acids (Omega 6's) are essential fatty acids that have a number of body functions. Along with omega-3 fatty acids, omega 6-fatty acids play a critical role in healthly brain function and normal growth and development. While omega-3 fatty acids tend to decrease inflammation, omega-6 fatty acids tend to promote it and may play a role in complex regional pain syndrome. Ideally the body should have a 1:1 ratio of omega-3 and omega-6 fatty acids from the diet. Omega-6's are found in eggs, cereals, fried foods, meats, poultry and some vegetable oils, including corn, grape seed, soybean, sunflower, and wheat germ oil.

Phytosterols are plant sterols with structures that are similar to cholesterol and in fact, inhibit the intestinal absorption of cholesterol and serum cholesterol. They have protective and disease-fighting benefits. Foods with the highest concentration of phytosterols include almonds, Brussels sprouts, canola oil, corn oil, macadamia nuts, olive oil, peanuts, rice bran oil, rye bread, sesame oil, wheat bran, and wheat germ.

Polyunsaturated fatty acids have many bonds that are unsaturated so they can easily be broken down by the body. This is not always a good feature since this may lead to instability, particularly when they are located within cellular membranes. Foods with higher amount of polyunsaturated fats include corn oil, fish (such as albacore tuna, herring, mackerel, salmon and trout), safflower, soybean, and sunflower oils, and walnuts.

Saturated fatty acids are fully saturated, which means that their bonds are filled. This feature normally makes them difficult for the body to break down, or metabolize. Generally saturated fatty acids are found in animal foods and beverages; however, coconut and palm oils are noted for their saturated fatty acid content.

Sterols (also known as steroid alcohols) are a type of steroid that occur naturally in animals (such as cholesterol), fungi and plants (such as phytosterols that are found in soy foods). Cholesterol is vital to animal cell membranes. It also functions as a precursor for making fat-soluble vitamins (vitamins A, D, E and K) and steroid hormones. Dietary cholesterol also contributes to increased risks of cardiovascular disease when it is elevated in blood cholesterol. Phytosterols, or plant sterols, have been shown to block cholesterol absorption and help to reduce serum cholesterol.

Trans fatty acids are of two kinds: naturally-occurring and artificial. Naturally occurring trans fatty acids are formed in the gut of some animals and foods (such as milk and meat products). Artificial trans fatty acids are created during industrial processes that add hydrogen using trans bonds to solidify liquid vegetable oils. Trans fatty acids were used in the U.S. because they were easy to use, inexpensive and long lasting. However, trans fatty acids raise LDL ("bad") cholesterol and lower HLD ("good") cholesterol and increase the risks of developing cardiovascular disease, type 2 diabetes, and stroke. In 2015, the U.S. Food and Drug Administration required that synthetic trans fatty acids be phased out of all foods within three years.

Triglycerides are the main form of lipids that are found in the body and in foods and beverages. Triglycerides are composed of a backbone molecule of glycerol (a sugar alcohol) and three fatty acids that can be saturated,

unsaturated or both. High serum triglycerides are associated with increased risks of cardiovascular disease and strokes and conditions such as hypothyroidism, kidney or liver ailments, metabolic syndrome, obesity, and uncontrolled type 2 diabetes may also be associated with elevated serum triglycerides. By eliminating alcohol, limiting dietary cholesterol and some saturated fats, losing weight, reducing simple carbohydrates, and restricting trans fatty acid intake, the serum triglyceride level may decrease.

Unsaturated fatty acids have one or more of their bonds that are unsaturated, which means that they are not filled. This is generally a good feature since the body can break down and metabolize unsaturated fatty acids more easily. Almonds, avocadoes, flax seeds, hazel nuts, macadamia nuts, peanut butter, salmon, sardines, seeds, vegetable oils, and walnuts contain unsaturated fatty acids.

How Coconuts Compare

The cardiovascular benefits of coconuts are revealed when each of these fats and oils are compared to the types of fats in coconuts. A comparison of raw coconuts, coconut oil, and coconut water follow:

Cholesterol (High-Density or HDL, Low-density or LDL and Very-low Density or VLDL)

• Since coconuts are from the plant kingdom, raw coconut, coconut oil, and coconut water do not contain any form of cholesterol.

Fats

• One cup of raw coconut contains 26.8 grams of total fat that are mostly saturated (23.8 grams compared to 26.8 grams total).

• One cup of coconut oil contains 218 grams of total fat that are mostly saturated (189 grams compared to 218 grams total).

• One cup of coconut water contains virtually no total fat (0.5 grams per one cup) or saturated fat (0.4 grams per one cup).

Hydrogenation

• Since hydrogenation is a process of converting unsaturated fatty acids into more saturated fatty acids, coconuts in their raw state do not contain hydrogenated fatty acids.

• Hydrogenated coconut oil

 - A small portion of the unsaturated fatty acids in coconut oil may be hydrogenated in order to keep the coconut oil solid at higher temperature. Outside of the US, hydrogenated and partially hydrogenated coconut oils may be used in the confection industry in baked goods or candies in tropical climates.

Lecithin

• Lecithin may be combined with coconut as an emulsifier; however, coconut oil with its higher concentration of saturated fatty acids is already semi- to fully solidified.

Lipids

• Because lipids are fats and oils, the fats that are found in coconuts are considered lipids.

• Since there is virtually not any total fat or saturated fat in one cup of coconut water, it does not significantly contain any lipids.

Oils

• Coconut oil can be extracted from raw coconut meat. The extraction rate may be as much as 75 percent.

• Coconut oil is in a semi-solid state at room temperature.

Essential fatty acids

• Omega-3 fatty acids
  - There are no omega-3 fatty acids in one cup of raw, shredded coconut, one cup of coconut oil or one cup of coconut water.

• Omega 6 fatty acids
  - There are 293 milligrams of omega-6 fatty acids in 1-cup of raw, shredded coconut.

  - There are 3,923 milligrams of omega-6 fatty acids in 1 cup of coconut oil.

  - There are 4.8 milligrams of omega-6 fatty acids in 1-cup of coconut water.

Phospholipids

• Phospholipids may be present in coconut endosperm and coconut oil.

Sterols

• Phytosterols
  - There are 37.6 milligrams of phytosterols in one cup of raw, shredded coconut.

  - There are 187 milligrams of phytosterols in one cup of coconut oil.

  - There are virtually no phytosterols in one cup of coconut water.

Saturated fatty acids

• The saturated fatty acids in coconuts are lauric (C12), myristic (C14) and stearic (C17).

- There are 23.8 grams of saturated fatty acids in one cup of raw, shredded coconut.

- There are 189 grams of saturated fatty acids in one cup of coconut oil.

- There are virtually no saturated fatty acids (0.4 grams) in one cup of coconut water.

Trans fats

- There are no trans fatty acids in raw coconut, coconut oil or coconut water.

Trigylcerides

• The saturated fatty acids in coconuts are medium-chain triglycerides that are extracted from coconut meat into coconut oil.

Unsaturated fatty acids

• Monounsaturated fatty acids

- There are 1.1 grams of monounsaturated fatty acids in one cup of raw, shredded coconut.

- There are 12.6 grams of monounsaturated fatty acids in one cup of coconut oil.

- There are virtually zero grams of monounsaturated fatty acids in 1-cup of coconut water.

• Polyunsaturated fatty acids

- There are 0.3 grams of polyunsaturated fatty acids in one cup of raw, shredded coconut.

- There are 3.9 grams of polyunsaturated fatty acids in one cup of coconut oil.

- There are virtually zero grams of polyunsaturated fatty acids in one cup of coconut water.

Greek Roast Chicken

1 whole roasting chicken (4 to 5 pounds)

3 tablespoons refined coconut oil, divided

2 tablespoons chopped fresh rosemary, plus 2 sprigs

2 cloves garlic, minced

1 small lemon

1¼ teaspoons salt, divided

½ teaspoon black pepper, divided

1 can (about 14 ounces) chicken broth, divided

2 large sweet potatoes, peeled and cut into thick wedges

1 medium red onion, cut into ¼-inch wedges

1 pound fresh asparagus spears, trimmed

1. Preheat oven to 425°F. Place chicken, breast side up, in shallow roasting pan. Combine 2 tablespoons oil, chopped rosemary and garlic in small bowl; brush over chicken.

2. Grate 1 teaspoon peel from lemon; set aside. Cut lemon into quarters; squeeze juice over chicken and place rinds and rosemary sprigs in chicken cavity. Sprinkle ¾ teaspoon salt and ¼ teaspoon pepper over chicken. Pour 1 cup broth into bottom of roasting pan; roast 30 minutes.

3. Reduce oven temperature to 375°F. Arrange sweet potatoes and onion wedges around chicken. Drizzle emaining broth and 1 tablespoon oil over vegetables; roast 15 minutes.

4. Arrange asparagus spears in roasting pan. Sprinkle remaining ½ teaspoon salt and ¼ teaspoon pepper over vegetables. Roast 10 minutes or until chicken is cooked through (165°F) and vegetables are tender. Transfer chicken to cutting board. Tent with foil; let stand 10 to 15 minutes.

5. Sprinkle reserved lemon peel over chicken. Carve chicken and serve with vegetables and pan juices.

Makes 8 serving

Greek Roast Chicken uses coconut oil for basting whole chicken, with garlic and herbs, red onions and sweet potatoes for a flavorsome and wholesome roasted entrée that's equally delicious cold.

Fat to Fight Fat?

Coconut, even with its high total fat and saturated fat content, has actually been shown to help aid weight loss. In this chapter the various ways that the coconut may contribute to the fight against body fat are discussed in depth.

For example, the medium-chain triglycerides (MCTs) in coconut oil may actually help to *burn* body fat and boost metabolism. Coconut has been thought to help metabolize abdominal fat. This is especially encouraging since excess abdominal fat is a known risk for heart disease and diabetes among other health conditions.

While the fat in coconut may help weight loss, it is important to recognize that it has the same number of calories per gram (9 calories/gram) as any other dietary fat, so coconut still should be consumed in moderation. Yet there are still smart ways to incorporate coconuts into healthy diets without being too excessive.

Using coconut oil for cooking instead of canola or olive oil may result in a *thermogenic effect* within the body, which means that it may help increase metabolism and in turn, increase energy. While this amount of energy may be low, it still adds up. Even more, eating coconut can lead to feelings of satiety and reduced appetite. This may result in fewer calories consumed overall.

This chapter also touches on some of the properties of coconut water. Unlike coconut oil, coconut water is virtually fat-free; it's also low in calories and contains nutrients such as vitamin C and potassium. Coconut water can be used for hydration, especially in place of sugary sports drinks or soft drinks, which is very helpful when people try to lose weight healthfully.

Energy

Energy is the ability to do work. It is measured in *calories*. A *calorie* is a unit of energy that often refers to the calorie content of foods and beverages. A calorie produces heat—in fact, a calorie is defined as the amount of heat that is required to raise the temperature of one kilogram of water one degree Centigrade. In the human body, the process of burning calories to produce energy (and heat) increases one's metabolism.

Metabolism is the sum of all of the chemical and physical processes by which energy is created and made available for life. There are many factors that are involved in metabolism and whether a person metabolizes or burns food and beverages quickly or slowly.

Factors that lower metabolism include age, fasting, hormones, sleep, and starvation. As a person ages their metabolism slows down, as it does with severe dieting. Hormones produced by the thyroid gland may either increase or decrease metabolism. And too much sleep means that the body is less active; thus, metabolism may be slower while a person is sleeping.

Factors that raise metabolism include caffeine, fever, gender (male), growth, height, lean body mass, nicotine, and stress. When a person is young, their metabolism is generally high. Gender-wise, taller and more muscular men tend to have a higher metabolism than shorter, rounder women.

Energy-producing nutrients (carbohydrates, lipids, and proteins) also affect metabolism; their effect depends on whether or not they are consumed and in what forms and combinations. As a type of lipid with very distinctive properties, coconut oil and its metabolism into energy can actually contribute to fat loss if used properly. However, do keep in mind that consuming any nutrient in excess may lead to weight gain.

Calories from Nutrients

The energy-producing nutrients each provide a distinct number of calories per gram when they are metabolized. Carbohydrates (sugars and starches) and proteins each yield about four calories per gram (4 calories/gram) while fats and oils each yield about nine calories per gram (9 calories/gram)—about twice as much as carbohydrates or proteins. This is why fats and oils are considered to be so caloric and "fattening".

Alcohol, while not a nutrient, contains seven calories per gram (7 calories/gram) and is metabolized as a fat, which is why regular alcohol consumption may also contribute to weight gain.

Weight Loss Strategies

In order to lose weight, a person needs to eat and drink less, exercise more, or some combination of both of these approaches. There must be a caloric deficit for weight loss. Conversely, if more calories are consumed rather than expended, weight will probably be gained.

There are many dietary strategies to accomplish weight loss including gluten-free, high-carbohydrate, high-fiber, high-protein, low-calorie, low-carbohydrate, and countless other approaches, programs, products, and potions. The use of coconut oil with its medium-chain triglycerides may have advantages. To understand how the medium-chain triglycerides that are found in coconuts contribute to weight loss, one must first understand more about fat digestion and metabolism.

Fat Digestion and Metabolism

The digestion of *lipids* (fats and oils) first begins in the mouth, where it is mostly physical. The teeth tear apart fat from other foods and the mouth begins to melt some of the fats. Then the residue passes through the esophagus into the stomach where it is mixed with stomach acid and water and some fat is broken down by the acid.

The process of breaking down lipids into its components of *triglycerides* with their fatty acids and *glycerol* is slow. Since lipids have so many calories per gram, they tend to stay around the stomach longer and may lead to satiety or fullness.

Once the triglyceride remnants pass into the small intestine, the smallest fatty acids (or short-chain fatty acids) and glycerol are able to pass through the intestinal wall into the bloodstream where they are transported to the liver, stored, or converted into other substances.

Longer-chain triglycerides (LCTs) are broken down by bile in the small intestine. *Bile* is an emulsifier that is made in the liver and stored in the gallbladder. It mixes with lipids along with watery digestive secretions and readies the lipids for additional breakdown by intestinal enzymes.

Medium-chain triglycerides (MCTs) have a different fate. For one, they are more easily metabolized than longer-chain triglycerides and may help to burn calories and support weight loss. Medium-chain triglycerides passively diffuse from the gastro-intestinal (GI) tract through the portal system to the liver without needing to be broken down, nor the necessity for bile salts for their digestion.

Since medium-chain triglycerides do not require energy for absorption, use, or storage they may be used in some infant formulas and nourishing supplements for hospitalized patients with fatty-acid metabolism disorders, malabsorption, or malnutrition.

Medium-chain triglycerides either do not affect total cholesterol nor raise HDL-cholesterol and they may also improve the ratio of LDL to HDL-cholesterol (LDL:HDL). Medium-chain triglycerides are also thought to promote quick fat oxidation. This is why some endurance athletes and body builders seem to favor MCTs. However, claims and conclusive results about their effectiveness seem to be mixed.

Besides all of these applications, medium-chain triglycerides may also have the potential to promote weight loss by increasing the metabolism. To fully comprehend why, an understanding of ketosis, particularly for weight loss, is essential.

Ketosis for Weight Loss

Ketogenic diets have been used for fast (and in some cases continued) weight loss for centuries. Ketogenic diets are also said to show promising results for epilepsy and neurodegenerative disorders, such as Alzheimer's and Parkinson's diseases, as discussed in Chapter 6.

First of all, let's answer a basic question: what is ketosis? Normally the human body uses glucose for energy. *Glucose* is a simple sugar that is the building block of carbohydrates (sugars and starches). When the human body metabolizes carbohydrates, they break down into glucose that can be used for energy or stored for future energy needs. Consuming too many carbohydrates may lead to excess calories and this may progress to obesity.

When glucose is not available for energy, the human body turns to an "intermediary" state for its energy needs. This is called *ketosis* when the human body produces *ketones*, by-products that form when the body burns stored fat for energy.

Some higher-protein and fat and lower-carbohydrate diets rely upon ketosis for fat loss and decreased body weight. Long term and uncontrolled, ketosis may develop into a state called *acidosis* that may lead to coma or even death. Ketosis may also occur during prolonged starvation.

To comprehend why ketogenic diets work and how medium-chain triglycerides interplay, one must first understand the process of *lipolysis*. Like glycolysis and the breakdown of carbohydrates to produce energy, lipolysis is the breakdown of lipids to produce energy.

When the body needs energy and it calls upon its stored carbohydrates, it may also call upon its lipid stores within its cells—particularly when carbohydrates "run out" as in prolonged starvation or long-term exercise. Enzymes break down stored lipids; then fatty acids and glycerol (from triglycerides) are released into the blood stream. When these fatty acids reach the muscle cells they enter *mitochondria* of the cell, or the cell's powerhouse and energy is released.

As mentioned, lipids have the capacity of supplying twice the amount of energy than carbohydrates or protein (9 calories/gram compared to 4 calories/gram respectively). This is the reason why fats and oils are so calorie dense and also why ketogenic diets may lead to faster weight loss than simple calorie reduction or some other carbohydrate-based diets.

Coconut Shrimp with Pear Chutney

Coconut Shrimp with Pear Chutney blends coconut oil with jalapeno pepper for heat, shallot, ginger, pear and green onion with shredded, unsweetened coconut, curry powder, butter and shrimp for a mouthwatering taste of the tropics. This dish can even be topped with more shredded and toasted coconut for the flavor to really pop.

½ cup shredded unsweetened coconut

¾ teaspoon curry powder

½ teaspoon salt

3 tablespoons coconut oil or melted unsalted butter

1 pound large raw shrimp, peeled and deveined

Pear Chutney (recipe follows)

1. Prepare Pear Chutney; set aside. Preheat oven to 425°F. Spray baking sheet with non-stick cooking spray.

2. Combine coconut, curry powder and salt in shallow dish. Toss shrimp with oil or melted butter to coat. Dip shrimp in coconut mixture, pressing lightly to adhere. Place on prepared baking sheet.

3. Bake 4 minutes. Turn over; bake 2 minutes or until shrimp are pink and opaque. Serve with Pear Chutney.

Makes 4 servings

1 tablespoon coconut oil

1 jalapeño pepper*, seeded and minced

1 small shallot, minced

1 teaspoon grated fresh ginger

1 medium unpeeled ripe pear, cored and cut into ½-inch pieces

2 teaspoons cider vinegar

1 teaspoon packed brown sugar

⅛ teaspoon salt

1 tablespoon water, plus more if necessary

1 tablespoon chopped green onion

Jalapeño peppers can sting and irritate the skin, so wear rubber gloves when handling peppers and do not touch your eyes.

1. Heat oil in medium saucepan over low heat. Add jalapeño, shallot and ginger; cook and stir 3 minutes or until shallot is tender.

2. Add pear, vinegar, brown sugar and salt. Stir in water. Cover and cook over low heat 15 minutes or until pear is tender, adding additional 1 tablespoon water if mixture becomes dry. Stir in green onion; cook 1 minute. Cool completely.

Makes 2 cups

Medium-chain Triglycerides and Weight Loss

The saturated fatty acids that are found in coconut oil with their medium-chain triglycerides are shorter in length than longer-chain triglycerides and they are more water-soluble than some other oils. The body processes these medium-chain triglycerides differently than longer-chain triglycerides. Longer-chain triglycerides must be mixed with a substance called *bile* that is produced by the gallbladder and then assaulted by pancreatic enzymes. Medium-chain triglycerides do not require bile or pancreatic enzymes, so once they reach the small intestine they diffuse through its membrane into the blood stream where they are more directly routed to the liver, converted into ketones, and metabolized as fuel.

The liver also releases ketones back into the blood stream where they are carried throughout the body. In this manner, ketones may be used for energy by the brain. This is significant since the brain has a protective barrier called the *"blood-brain barrier"* that these ketones can cross.

As a result, ketones have fewer tendencies to be deposited in fat stores and more opportunities to be metabolized by the body for various purposes. Additionally, medium-chain triglycerides provide antioxidant, anti-inflammatory, and even anti-microbial functions inside the gut where they fight potentially harmful bacteria, fungi, parasites, and viruses.

Medium-chain Triglyceride Structures

Medium-chain triglycerides are distinguished by their carbon lengths:

• Caproic acid (C6) -6 carbons

• Caprylic acid (C8) – 8 carbons

• Capric acid (C10) – 10 carbons

• Lauric acid (C12) – 12 carbons

In general, the fewer number of carbon molecules, the shorter the chain and the easier and more efficiently that medium-chain triglycerides will converted into ketones for energy with less reactive oxygen that may be damaging to the body.

Coconut oil has a mixture of medium-chain fatty acids, with about 40 percent of it as *lauric acid*.

Some studies suggest that coconut oil with its medium-chain triglycerides and particularly lauric acid may help to reduce one's midsection, but that it may not contribute to improved body mass index (BMI) or significant weight loss.

The ketones also help to control the hormone *ghrelin*, the "hunger" hormone that is produced in the gastrointestinal tract. Ghrelin functions within the central nervous system to increase appetite. *Leptin*, the appetite "suppressor" hormone, controls ketone utilization in the neurons of the *hypothalamus* (the hunger control center of the brain) that helps to decreases one's appetite.

Medium-chain Triglycerides and Weight

It is known that medium-chain triglycerides may boost *thermogenesis* (heat production) and fat oxidation for energy and that both of these processes may suppress the accumulation of body fat. Another way that medium-chain triglycerides may help with weight loss efforts is by helping with appetite reduction.

Consuming foods and beverages with fat may turn off a desire to eat more calories because fats provide such concentrated calories. Even a little bit of fat that is consumed at meals has staying power.

There is also some speculation that medium-chain triglycerides act on other hormones that may include cholecystokinin, gastric inhibitory peptide, neurotensin, pancreatic polypeptide, and/or peptide YY. The exact modes of operation are unknown. However, it is speculated that these actions may help to decrease appetite and increase satiety.

The *body mass index* is a ratio of weight-to-height that is used to indicate obesity and underweight.

Coconut Oil and Calories

One tablespoon of coconut oil contains approximately 121 calories. Coconut oil is pretty similar in calories when compared to other oils. In comparison, one tablespoon of the following oils contain:

Type of oil	Calories per 1 Tablespoon
Almond oil	119
Avocado oil	124
Canola oil	124
Corn oil	124
Cottonseed oil	119
Extra-virgin olive oil	120
Flaxseed oil	119
Grapeseed oil	119
Hazelnut oil	119
Hemp seed oil	130
Macadamia oil	120
Olive oil	119
Palm oil	119
Palm kernel oil	116
Peanut oil	119
Safflower oil	119
Sesame oil	119
Soybean oil	119
Sunflower oil	119
Vegetable oil	120
Walnut oil	119
Wheat germ oil	119

It is important to keep in mind that one tablespoon of coconut oil contains about 13.47 grams of total fat (almost all fat). So coconut oil is very calorie-dense, even in smaller quantities. While the medium-chain triglycerides in coconut oil do pass through the digestion, absorption, and metabolism quicker than other oils and fats, consuming too much coconut oil or other oil may lead to extra calories.

Use of Medium-chain Triglycerides by Endurance Athletes

Coconut oil has been valued for its relationship to weight and energy expenditure among endurance athletes. Coconut oil supplies energy; it has the capability to support fitness since it may boost energy, enhance performance, and support endurance. Also, coconut oil may improve the digestion and absorption of nutrients—especially those that require a little fat for their digestion and assimilation. And coconut oil is thought to assist in blood sugar utilization and insulin secretion. Suggested dosages vary.

Since medium-chain triglycerides are digested easier than longer triglycerides, the thought is that they may help to increase energy metabolism during both medium and high-intensity exercise. Medium-chain triglycerides helped to reduce the body's reliance on carbohydrates as a fuel for exercise and decrease the amount of *lactate* that is produced during exercise that may lead to increased endurance.

High lactate levels increase the acidity of the muscle cells and disrupt other metabolites. Metabolic pathways perform poorly within this type of acidic environment. This is a natural defense mechanism of the body to help prevent permanent damage during extreme exertion by slowing down key systems to help maintain muscle contraction. Then oxygen becomes more available and metabolism can continue for energy and recovery from strenuous exercise. Medium-chain triglycerides may help to prevent or reduce these processes from occurring.

Disadvantages of Medium-chain Triglycerides

Medium-chain triglycerides may induce *ketogenesis* (the release of ketones by the body when fats are broken down for energy) and *metabolic acidosis* (a condition that occurs when the body produces too much acid or when the kidneys are not removing enough acid from the body). Under certain conditions, ketogenesis may be desirable. However, metabolic acidosis may lead to shock or death.

If medium-chain triglycerides are consumed in high quantities they may provoke gastrointestinal side effects including loose stools.

Coconut Water, Weight, and Sports Performance

Coconut water is virtually fat-free and low in calories with some nutrients including vitamin C and potassium. It can be used for hydration to replace sugary sports drinks or soft drinks, which is important for people who try to lose weight and for athletes to remain healthy while they train and compete.

A comparison of water, coconut water, sports drinks, and soft drinks shows the advantages and disadvantages of these fluids.

Water is a fluid of choice for everyday consumption and for everyday exercise. For exercise that is greater in duration or intensity, or for exercisers who heavily perspire, some fluids may be better for hydration. Some brands of sports drinks and coconut water with potassium may be effective for muscle cramps.

Coconut water is also a natural way to add potassium, hydrate, and reduce sodium in everyday diets that reply upon sports drinks as regular beverages. This is because coconut water has fewer calories and less sodium than some sports drinks. Also, many Americans do not obtain enough potassium in their daily diets from dairy products or fresh fruits and vegetables, so coconut water may help to provide some needed nutrients.

When a person exercises strenuously in excess of three hours (as the time expended in a marathon) and they sweat heavily, they will probably need easily absorbable carbohydrates for energy (such as the sugar that is found in sports drinks), as well as electrolytes such as potassium and sodium. This is why unsweetened coconut water may be limiting in its use for hydration and sports drinks may be more satisfying and hydrating under extreme conditions.

An option during hot weather events or practice might be to mix coconut water with a little salt. Coconut water with added sodium may be better tolerated than some sports drinks post-exercise and may not cause as much fullness, stomach upset, or nausea as some report.

Some athletes may choose to drink coconut water the evening before an intense workout or event—especially during difficult heat conditions.

One concern about the use of coconut water for exercise is whether or not the amount of coconut water consumed replenishes what the body loses during exercise. A simple test is the color of urine that should be clear. It is important to note that taste matters when it comes to replacing body fluids. So if athletes enjoy the taste of coconut water and are able to consume coconut water in adequate amounts, then it might be more efficient for hydration than water.

Coconut water may be combined with protein powder to help the muscles recover after an event or heavy workout. In either case, the use of coconut water before, during, or after heavy exercise or under extreme conditions should first be tested during practice. Athletic trainers and coaches may also provide advice.

Comparison of Calories

A comparison of calories, carbohydrates, fat, and protein in water, coconut water, sports drinks, fruit juice, and cola follow:

- **Tap and non-mineralized water (per 1 fluid ounce)**

   - Zero calories, zero carbohydrates, zero fat, zero protein

- **Unflavored coconut water (per 1 fluid ounce)**

   - 5.45 calories, 1.3 grams sugar, 61 milligrams (mg) potassium 5.45 milligrams mg sodium

- **Sports drinks (per 1 fluid ounce)**

   - 6.25 calories, 1.75 grams sugar, 3.75 milligrams (mg) potassium, 13.75 milligrams (mg) sodium

- **Fruit juice (per 1 fluid ounce)**

   - 3.9 calories, 2.6 grams sugar, 62 milligrams (mg) potassium, 0.3 milligrams (mg) sodium

- **Cola (per 1 fluid ounce)**

   - 11.3 calories, 2.7 grams sugar, 0.6 milligrams (mg) potassium, 1.2 milligrams (mg) sodium

Coconut Water for Weight Management

Consuming a liquid before a meal may cause one to eat less. This is the theory behind a "slow-up liquid". A slow-up liquid can be sipped before a meal, with or without ice and a flavorful herb or fruit slice to boost the flavor.

Try coconut water with a sprig of basil, mint, or parsley or a spear of cucumber, jicama, or fennel. The calories are fairly negligible. It may seem and look like a cocktail, refresh, and help to mitigate the ravishing feeling some may feel right before a meal.

To add the flavor of coconut water to beverages without packing on calories, try freezing coconut water in an ice cube tray, then adding a few cubes to perk up the flavor of ordinary water. The taste will be appealing without overwhelming and may be enjoyed by those who do not enjoy a stronger coconut taste.

For those people who can afford more calories, but prefer to avoid commercial sports drinks, mixing one-half coconut water with one-half fruit juice provides a fuller fruit taste with half of the calories than a full glass of fruit juice. Plus, there is more potassium along with varying amounts of choline, folate, vitamins A, C, calcium, magnesium, and phosphorus depending upon the type of coconut water that is used.

Coconut water also has many applications in cooking and baking. It can be used in some recipes in place of a few teaspoons of water, but keep in mind its sweet taste. In some recipes, coconut water will enhance the sweetness. In other recipes, it may quash the bitterness. And in other recipes, the sweet taste might be tamed by a touch of salt, which may even taste tropical.

A little bit of natural fruit or vegetable juice can be added to coconut water for additional color, taste, natural sugar. and some vitamins and minerals.

Speaking of the tropics, coconut water may be an excellent addition to some Asian or Caribbean recipes because of its natural affinity to the tropical fruits and vegetables in these recipes, but it may also lend a sweet and tasty touch to marinades, sauces, or even soups. It contributes the coconutty taste without the heaviness of coconut oil. In addition, coconut water can be used in some recipes along with coconut oil and even grated coconut.

Coconut Melon Water Smoothie

- **6 ounces frozen coconut water (about 6 ice cubes made from coconut water)***
- **1 cup cubed melon (cantaloupe, honeydew or watermelon)**
- **1 tablespoon citrus zest (lemon, lime or orange)**
- **Mint leaf, to garnish**

Coconut water can be frozen in an ice cube tray. This recipe requires about six coconut water ice cubes; however size and number may vary depending upon the ice cube tray.

1. Combine the first three ingredients into a blender.

2. Blend until smooth, frothy consistency.

3. Garnish with mint. If a minty flavor preferred, mint leaf can be blended with other ingredients.

> *Makes about 1⅔ cups, depending upon the size of the ice cubes.*

Use Your Brain

Some of the more interesting research that surrounds the healing power of coconut involves the possible links between coconut oil and decreased dementia and epilepsy. Much of this research surrounds the ketogenic diet: a diet that higher in fat and lower in carbohydrates than is generally recommended, which forces the body to burn fat for fuel.

This chapter describes the ketogenic diet in detail, how coconuts may fit into ketogenic diets, and why ketogenic diets may be beneficial for certain disorders. For example, the ketogenic diet has been shown to be effective at reducing seizures in children

with epilepsy. This discovery has led scientists to theorize that coconut oil may be useful for people with Alzheimer's disease and dementia.

This chapter also describes methods by which the coconut may prevent general aging in the brain and help improve memory.

Ketogenic Diets

The *ketogenic diet* has been used for a variety of disorders since the 1920s when it was designed by Dr. Russell Wilder at the Mayo Clinic in Rochester, Minnesota, as a treatment for epilepsy. After anti-seizure medications came to the forefront in the 1940s, the ketogenic diet somewhat lost its appeal. While low-carbohydrate, ketogenic-like diets have a long history, they became popularized in the US in the late 1960s to early 1970s when the Stillman and Atkins diets first became popularized. Their premise is pretty much the same: the process of ketosis could effectively be employed for weight loss.

The premise of ketogenic diets is that with higher-fat, adequate protein, and low carbohydrates the body is forced into "burning" its stored body fats for energy rather than carbohydrates, the preferred energy source.

Under "normal" conditions, the human body digests and metabolizes the carbohydrates that are contained in foods and beverages and converts them into glucose for energy. Glucose is then transported to many various body cells and also fuels the brain.

When there are few carbohydrates available, then the liver is capable of converting fat into fatty acids and *ketone bodies*, molecules that can also be oxidized for energy. These ketones bodies can then pass through the *brain barrier* (a highly selective semipermeable membrane that protects the brain) and replace glucose as a source of energy. When ketones are elevated in the blood it may result in a state of ketosis that has both advantages but also disadvantages.

The advantages of ketosis are that it can be used as a medical intervention for diabetes or epilepsy, endurance exercise, or significant weight loss. Ketogenic diets may reduce hunger and lower overall food intake that may be particularly effective in reating the severely obese.

The disadvantages of ketosis are that it may alter blood lipid levels (both positively and negatively), lead to fatigue, stress the kidneys, trigger micronutrient deficiencies, and instigate ketoacidosis which could be fatal at extremes for diabetics.

Epilepsy

Fasting to treat disease has been a topic of discourse since ancient Greek and Indian physicians utilized it in their practices. An early treatise in the Hippocratic Corpus "On the Sacred Disease" (supposedly written in 400 BC) describes how dietary alterations may affect epilepsy management—particularly in the abstinence of food and drink.

Because of the potential dangers of it, any use of ketogenic diets, particularly for children, should first be reviewed with a health care practitioner.

The first study that examined fasting as an epileptic treatment occurred in France in 1911. Patients were placed on a low-calorie vegetarian diet instead of receiving the treatment of the time, potassium bromide. While potassium bromide curbed the epileptic seizures it also reportedly lowered the mental capacity of the study subjects. The diet plus fasting led to improved mental capabilities.

Three main ketone bodies were at the forefront of diabetes research in the 1920s. When otherwise healthy people were starved or consumed a very low-carbohydrate, high-fat diet, then a higher level of these ketone bodies were produced. This higher level of serum (blood) ketones is referred to as *ketonemia*.

Subsequently, anticonvulsant treatments were used to treat epilepsy. Still, epileptic control was not fully achieved. The ketogenic diet was later reintroduced as a therapy to treat children with epilepsy. After an 18 to 25 day fast some children became seizure free; others showed some improvement, while still other children demonstrated the most success on what was referred to as a "water diet". The idea of fasting subsequently became a conventional treatment for epilepsy along with abidying by dietary carbohydrate restriction.

Weight Loss

The use of ketone bodies has also been used for dieting nearly as long as they have been used to treat epilepsy.

In the 1920s, an endocrinologist detected that ketone bodies, produced by the liver as a side effect of fasting or a diet that was high in fat and low in carbohydrates, were effective for weight loss. This type of dietary approach became known as the low-carbohydrate/ketogenic diet. It has had many guises throughout the years. Some of the books that recommended it included the 1958 book *Eat Fat and Grow Slim* by Dr. Richard Mackarness; the 1967 book *The Doctor's Quick Weight Loss Diet* by Dr. Irwin Stillman; and the 1972 book *Dr. Atkins Diet Revolution.*

The later Zone, Paleo, and Dukan diets base their diet strategies and successes on the fundamentals of ketosis.

Ketogenic diets may contain 70 percent or more daily calories from fat; five to 10 percent of total daily calories from carbohydrates (about 20 to 50 grams daily); and the remaining calories from proteins. Some more conservative dietary approaches are higher in carbohydrates (45 to 65 percent of total calories), lower in fat (20 to 35 percent of total calories), and moderate in protein (10 to 35 percent of total calories). Since 1980 and every five years thereafter, the U.S. Dietary Guidelines for Americans were published with renditions of these dietary approaches, which are now less specific in nature.

In order to adhere to a ketogenic diet with these nutritional parameters, one needs to greatly reduce or eliminate carbohydrate-containing foods such as dairy products, fruit, grains, legumes, and starchy vegetables. High protein foods such as eggs, fish, shellfish, meats, and poultry are the mainstays with very-low calorie vegetables as fillers. Fats as butter and oils are also featured. Alcohol is not included.

Some studies show that weight loss may be greater on a ketogenic diet than on a diet that is simply reduced in calories. Other studies indicate that the average weight loss after one year on a ketogenic diet may be greater than a low-fat diet and that serum triglycerides and blood pressure may decrease while high-density lipoproteins (HDL or "good" cholesterol) may increase. Even if weight loss stabilizes, after a few years high-density lipoproteins may continue to improve on a ketogenic diet. Like many diets, weight loss slows as a result of the body acclimating to its dietary parameters.

Blackberry Lime Smoothie

- ½ **cup unsweetened coconut milk**
- 1 **cup fresh blackberries**
- 2 **ice cubes**
- 1 **tablespoon fresh lime juice**
- 2 **teaspoons honey**
- ½ **teaspoon grated lime peel**

Combine coconut milk, blackberries, ice, lime juice, honey and lime peel in blender; blend until smooth. Serve immediately.

Blackberry Lime Smoothie is a super purple blend of coconut milk, blackberries, ice cubes, fresh lime juice, honey and grated lime peel. Blackberries are good sources of vitamins A, C, K and K, the antioxidants lutein and zeaxanthin, minerals that include copper, folic acid, magnesium, manganese, niacin, potassium, pantothenic acid, pyridoxine, riboflavin, and insoluble and soluble fibers. And the coconut milk and lime create a refreshing and nutritious tropical snack treat.

Positive Aspects of Ketogenic Diets

Meat has been a significant foundation of the U.S. diet, especially post World War II when it has been associated with prosperity. Aside from economics, meat is very satisfying with its fat content and robust taste. It has a very primeval appeal since its protein content is essential for life. Both prehistoric and modern people have sought meat for its amino acids—the staff of life. The ketogenic diet, with its high reliance on meat, is no exception.

In terms of the high fat content of ketogenic diets, fat is a concentrated source of energy with nine calories per gram. Prehistoric people were forced to eat when food was abundant and few parts of animals were left behind. Fat provided the staying power for days at end until the next capture or catch. In modern times fat still is very satisfying for hours on end—sometimes up to nine hours. Satiety from fat may prevent people from scrounging around for sugar- and calorie-filled foods and beverages.

Calorie counting (and often portion control) is not required in some ketogenic diets. This aspect may be very appealing to people who do not have the time nor the interest in doing it.

Perhaps one of the most important features of ketogenic diets is the lack of hunger. This is because ketone bodies tend to lower the level of *ghrelin* in the body. Ghrelin is a hormone that decreases hunger and promotes satiety. This is especially important between meals to help to manage appetite control.

The weight loss on a ketogenic diet may be more rapid than in a reduced-calorie or reduced-fat diet. This phenomenon may be very appealing to dieters because initial weight loss may be very motivational to continue dieting. When carbohydrates are limited as they are on a ketogenic diet, the body turns to its carbohydrates stores in the muscles and to liver glycogen. The initial weight loss on a ketogenic diet tends to be mostly water weight because when stored

Per person, U.S. residents consume more meat than in any other country worldwide.

carbohydrates are broken down for energy, water is also released (glycogen is stored with water). After about two to three weeks of dieting, this water loss diminishes and fat loss increases, particularly when the diet is accompanied by exercise.

Protein, too, can be used for energy, but this is not the preferred fuel. The muscles, including the heart, are made of protein and these stores must be preserved. This is another benefit of ketogenic diets: most provide more than enough protein to help to "spare" the body's protein stores from use.

Another advantage of a ketogenic diet is its capability of improving serum triglyceride and high-density lipoproteins and potentially lowering the risk of cardiovascular disease. Diets of this nature are also capable of lowering the tendencies for elevated blood sugar, *C-reactive protein* (which is a sign of inflammation and a marker for certain degenerative diseases), insulin, and waist circumference.

Problems with Ketogenic Diets

Eating the same high fat and high protein foods and beverages day in and day out over time may become boring (like so many other diets), which may cause backsliding over time. Other criticisms of the ketogenic diet are that it narrows food choices, compromises nutrient intake, makes it difficult to eat out or socialize since alcohol and many desserts are prohibited, and may even lead to digestive issues.

Since the ketogenic diet is limited or void of carbohydrates with fibers (even fruits, vegetables, and whole grains), normal digestion and elimination might be compromised and a natural fiber supplement may be warranted.

Caution: Higher protein stores may tax the kidneys and the liver that are involved in processing and excreting the by-products of protein breakdown: urea, uric acid, ammonia.

It is important to keep the gastrointestinal tract and especially the colon healthy to protect against certain GI diseases and particularly against colon cancer.

Nutrient deficiencies may also be a concern on a ketogenic diet. Nutrients such as vitamins A, C, D, and thiamine and minerals such as calcium, magnesium, and selenium may be lacking and might require supplementation. A health professional should be consulted before trying any diet—particularly one long term. Children, pregnant and nursing mothers, and the elderly should take special care and caution.

Coconuts and Ketogenic Diets

Research on ketogenic diets from the 1960s demonstrated that more ketones are produced by medium chain triglycerides (MCTs) per unit of energy than other sources of energy. This is because medium-chain triglycerides are quickly transported to the liver via the hepatic portal vein as opposed to through the lymphatic system.

It follows that if a diet that is rich in medium-chain triglycerides but reduced in carbohydrates, then it might be effective in treating epilepsy and in weight control management. In fact, a diet with 60 percent medium-chain triglycerides with protein and some carbohydrates has been shown to provide more meal options for children with epilepsy. Dieters may also be able to tolerate fewer carbohydrates without boredom if a little variety is provided.

Coconut to the rescue! The range and depth of recipes and meals with coconut in all of its forms are mind boggling, but for ketogenic diets, coconut oil with its high medium-chain triglycerides are key. Some recommendations suggest taking one to three tablespoons of coconut oil or MCT oil that is made from coconut oil daily. But this practice should support a ketonic diet, not replace it.

The Aging Brain

The brain ages like all bodily systems, organs, muscles, nerves, and cells. Specific changes in the brain due to aging include changes in blood vessels, free radicals, inflammation, neurons and neurotransmitters, plaques, and tangles and shrinkage.

Blood vessels in the brain may be compromised because arteries narrow with aging and there is less growth of new capillaries that occur. This may result in less blood being able to circulate and nourish the brain.

Free radical damage from cigarette smoke, herbicides, pollution, radiation, and a host of other environmental factors may accumulate with age. Free radicals are normally made in the mitochondria inside cells. They help the body's immune system to fight bacteria and viruses. However, free radicals may also damage the cell membranes of neurons or their DNA. This may instigate a chain reaction that releases more free radicals and cause further neurological damage.

Cells and compounds that are known to be involved in inflammation have been located in Alzheimer's Disease plaques, so it is thought that inflammation may have a role in the disease. Inflammation increases when the body responds to abnormal situations, disease, injuries, or even stress.

Other changes in the brain are the result of changes in the neurons and neurotransmitters that are responsible for communications among neurons. If and when the white matter of the brain is reduced, then communication among neurons may be compromised.

Keep in mind that each tablespoon of coconut oil contains about 117 calories and MCT oil about 100 calories and while calories do not necessarily need to be counted on a ketogenic diet, they may add up substantially.

Different parts of the brain actually shrink during aging, particularly the *prefrontal cortex* at the front of the frontal lobe and the *hippocampus*. Both vital to complex mental activities including learning, memory, and planning.

Structures referred to as *amyloid plaques* and *neurofibrillary tangles* develop both inside and outside of the neurons. *Amyloid plaques* contain largely insoluble deposits of seemingly toxic protein fragments. It is not conclusive whether these plaques cause Alzheimer's Disease or whether they are by-products of the disease.

Neurofibrillary tangles are abnormal collections of twisted protein threads within the nerve cells that contain phosphate molecules. These threads may become so enmeshed that they may become tangled within the cells, disrupt the healthy neuron transport network, and damage neuron communication.

Decreased brain glucose metabolism has been identified before the onset of clinically measurable cognitive decline and may contribute to further cascading decline. The process of aging appears to increase the risks of deteriorating glucose utilization in some regions of the brain.

Alzheimer's Disease

Alzheimer's disease (AD) is a progressive neurodegenerative disorder that primarily affects the elderly, but can impact earlier in life. There are two types of Alzheimer's disease: *early* and *late-onset*. Early onset Alzheimer's disease may strike a person early as their 30s, while late onset Alzheimer's disease may strike a person in their 70s or 80s and is the leading cause of dementia in people over 65 years of age. At the onset, people might experience memory loss and disorientation. As the disease progresses, additional cognitive functions may become impaired.

While there are theories that try to describe the course of the events that lead to Alzheimer's disease, the complete picture remain unknown. There are no totally effective prevention methods or treatments for Alzheimer's disease; however, there are some drugs that act as acetylcholinesterase inhibitors. *Acetylcholinesterase* is an enzyme that serves to terminate synaptic nerve transmission. These drugs enhance the effectiveness of nerve cells that are still functional but do not address the underlying pathology of Alzheimer's disease.

Dementia

Dementia covers a wide range of symptoms that are associated with a decline in memory and/or other skills that are involved in everyday activities. Alzheimer's disease is one form of dementia; it is estimated to account for about 60 to 80 percent of the instances of dementia. Another prominent type of dementia, *vascular dementia*, may occur after a stroke. Other conditions that may contribute to dementia are thyroid problems and vitamin deficiencies.

Signs of dementia may include the decreased ability to focus and pay attention; changes in memory, judgment, and reasoning; communication and language issues; and visual perception alterations. However, other environmental and physical factors may contribute to these signs of dementia.

Memory

Many cells in the body are formed and decline over a person's lifetime. Neurons develop throughout a person's life, but the brain reaches its maximum potential of neurons during a person's early 20s. They then slowly begin to decline in volume. Blood flow to the brain also decreases over time. However, the brain is capable of regrowth and learning and retaining new facts and skills. The more active that a person is, the more frequently their brain is stimulated. The better nourished that a person is, the better the odds that their brain will function well throughout their senior years.

Both episodic and long-term memory decline over time, as well as information processing and learning new information, doing more than one task at a time, and shifting focus to new tasks.

Coconuts in Ketogenic Diets and Brain Health

Coconuts with their medium-chain triglycerides have been associated with improved cognition and a number of enhanced brain functions. Studies have not definitively shown that medium-chain triglycerides can prevent dementia, but people with dementia might discover some short-term benefits by incorporating the medium-chain triglycerides like those that are found in coconuts into their diets.

Small clinical trials in aging individuals that had age-related cognitive decline and diabetic patients have shown that an MCT supplement can preserve cognitive function or lead to cognitive improvement. Medium-chain triglyceride supplementation appeared to help the diabetic patients but not the aging group.

Insulin, the hormone that regulates blood sugar, has been linked to changes in the brain that have been associated with Alzheimer's disease. This is the reason why this study was conducted with diabetic patients. It is not exactly clear what role insulin has in Alzheimer's disease. Furthermore, changes in the brain that are associated with dementia may be unconnected to glucose metabolism.

Memory problems may be exacerbated by factors such as anxiety, dehydration, depression, infection, medications, nutrition, stress, substance abuse, or thyroid imbalance.

Medium-chain triglyceride supplements also have been shown to improve cognitive function in people with mild cognitive impairment and Alzheimer's disease. A few studies suggest some cognition improvement and prevention of amyloid plaque formation in animals but human studies have not been confirmed.

A recent study suggested that although the effects of coconut oil may be temporary, that both Alzheimer's and dementia patients had some short-term benefits from supplementation. Another study that examined the effects of a mild ketogenic diet during exercise, both with and without ketosis, demonstrated that endurance and cognitive function were both increased.

There is strong evidence that exists that the use of medium-chain triglycerides by healthy adults is considered to be low risk. Foods and beverages, such as coconut oil, that are high in medium-chain triglycerides have been widely used with few reported adverse reactions.

The medium-chain triglycerides with lauric acid in organic, cold-pressed, non-hydrogenated virgin coconut oil, which make up nearly 60 percent of the total fat content of coconut oil are preferable. For comparison: one tablespoon of coconut oil contains about 7.4 grams of MCTs; butter contains about 1 gram of MCTs; and palm kernel oil contains about 7.9 grams of MCTs.

In some clinical studies, 10 to 40 grams (0.4 to 1.4 ounces) of medium-chain triglycerides are ingested daily, although some reports indicate that a daily dose up to about 70 grams of medium-chain triglycerides may produce demonstrable results. Mild gastrointestinal side effects may be common in some individuals who consume medium-chain triglycerides. These side effects may be offset by consuming medium-chain triglycerides with food and by slowly incorporating MCTs into one's diet. Like other supplements or medications, it is important to discuss the usage of MCT's with a health care provider before executing.

Butternut Squash Oven Fries are a take off on popular sweet potato fries. Butternut squash is rich in vitamin A, beta-carotene (a vitamin A precursor) and folate, niacin, potassium, riboflavin, pantothenic acid, thiamin, Vitamin B6, and fiber. Plus, the combination of butternut squash with coconut oil is so richly and sweetly satisfying that one hardly needs dessert!

Butternut Squash Oven Fries

½ **teaspoon garlic powder**

¼ **teaspoon salt**

¼ **teaspoon ground red pepper**

1 **butternut squash (about 2½ pounds), peeled, seeded and cut into thin 2-inch-long sticks**

1 **tablespoon coconut oil**

1. Preheat oven to 425°F. Combine garlic powder, salt and red pepper in small bowl.

2. Place squash on baking sheet. Drizzle with oil and sprinkle with seasoning mix; gently toss to coat. Arrange in single layer.

3. Bake 20 to 25 minutes or until squash just begins to brown, stirring frequently.

4. Preheat broiler. Broil 3 to 5 minutes or until fries are browned and crisp. Spread on paper towels to cool slightly before serving.

Primary Considerations

A ketogenic diet must be followed very strictly because the body prefers glucose for metabolism. The simple addition of coconut oil to the diet may not necessarily provide the neurons in the brain with an alternative source for energy. The most optimal use of coconut oil for brain health may be its incorporation into a finely devised ketogenic diet. In this context, the rich concentration of medium-chain triglycerides in coconut oil will probably comprise a prescribed amount of the total daily fat intake and should be in the correct proportion to the amount of carbohydrates and proteins. An experienced dietitian/nutritionist or health care provider may be able to devise and monitor such a diet.

Things That Go Bump

Not only are coconuts valued for culinary uses, but their medicinal values are also impressive. Coconuts provide the natural substances that are used for the development of many medicinals. Coconuts have a long list of antibacterial, antifungal, antiviral, antiparasitic, antidermatophytic, antioxidant, hypoglycemic, hepatoprotective, and immunostimulant properties. That long list means that coconuts fight bacteria, funguses, viruses, and parasites! They also protect the cells, skin, liver, and immune system among other bodily parts and functions.

This chapter explores the many ways that coconuts can be used for minor bumps and bruises. The antimicrobial properties of coconut are described, plus how coconuts can be beneficial for a host of minor ailments. For instance, coconut oil may be used to sooth bee stings,

bug bites, and minor scrapes and scratches. Coconut oil may be applied as an insect repellant and reportedly may be used to prevent or treat lice infestation. When coconut oil is ingested, its antibacterial and antiviral properties may protect against common colds and even strengthen the immune system.

Medicinal Effects

The medicinal effects of coconuts are many and varied, due in great part to their concentration of medium-chain triglycerides and lauric acid that were discussed previously.

Coconuts contain microminerals and other nutrients that are essential to human health and are used as preventatives and curatives worldwide, mainly in the tropics.

Of late, coconuts have been touted for their antiatherosclerotic, antibacterial, anticancer, anticarie, anticholecystic, antidermatophytic, antidote, antidiabetic, antifungal, antioxidant, antiprotozoal, antithrombic, antiviral, cardio-protective, electrolyte, hepatroprotective, hormone-like, hypolipidemic, and immunostimulatorie effects. The following conditions have been recounted, though many have not been thoroughly supported by extensive scientific research.

• **Antiatherosclerotic:** A coconut oil-based diet that is high in saturated fatty acids, particularly lauric acid and monolaurin acid, may lower antigen concentrations and may favorably affect lipoproteins, considered heart-healthy. This is in comparison to diets that are higher in mono- or polyunsaturated fatty acids.

• **Antibacterial:** Around the world, virgin coconut water is used to treat *cholera* (an infectious and sometimes fatal disease of the small intestine), diarrhea, and urinary tract infections, due to its saline and albumen content. The medium-chain triglyceride lauric acid in coconuts may also be effective at destroying lipid-coated bacteria that may lead to dental cavities, food poisoning, sinusitis, stomach ulcers, and urinary tract infections.

• **Anticancer:** Coconut husk fibers may be a source of drugs that work to overcome cancer resistance and promote tumor cell death.

• **Anticarie:** A coconut-based mouthwash that is made with coconut tree roots may be used as a gargle and mouthwash. Coconut extract may have potential in the prevention and treatment of oral disease. Coconut flour with its antimicrobial properties from lauric acid has been used for some oral infections that include mouth sores. And the compound sucrose monolaurate in coconuts may have anti-caries benefits by helping to prevent dental plaque. There is more about coconuts and oral health in Chapter 9.

• **Anticholecystic:** Coconuts may act as an urinary antiseptic and be effective in the treatment of kidney and urethral stones. They may be 50 to 75 percent effective in dissolving gallstones, due to the compound monoctanoin from the caprylic acid that is one of the three fatty acids that are contained within coconuts.

• **Antidermatophytic:** Coconut oil is used worldwide for its antiseptic effect and as a skin moisturizer. It may selectively combat bacteria and proactively treat atopic dermatitis.

• **Antidote:** Virgin coconut water is reported to eliminate poisons (as in the case of mineral poisoning) and improve drug-induced toxicity from over dosage.

• **Antidiabetic:** The coconut kernel may help to reverse the levels of glycogen in the body, the activities of carbohydrate metabolizing enzymes and pancreatic damage.

• **Antifungal:** Monolaurin and lauric acid in coconut oil may have an antifungal effect against spore germination and radical growth and may help to combat yeast overgrowth, such as candida and thrush.

• **Antioxidants:** The amino acid L-arginine and vitamin C in virgin coconut water may help to reduce damaging free radicals and lipid peroxidation.

• **Antiprotozoal:** Polyphenolic-rich coconuts may inhibit the growth of *protozoa* (microscopic organisms that flourish in moist environments and human parasites that cause diseases such as amoebic dysentery or malaria).

• **Antithromic:** Virgin coconut oil may lower antigen concentrations and may favorably affect the fibrinolytic system that is closely linked to control of inflammation and associated disease states.

Virgin coconut oil is reported to lower total cholesterol, phospholipids, triglycerides, low-density lipoproteins, and very-low-density lipoproteins and increase high-density lipoprotein cholesterol—all cardio-protective measures.

• **Antiviral:** Coconut oil may be effective against lipid-coated viruses that include Epstein-Barr, influenza, pneumono, hepatitis C, and CMV. The medium-chain triglycerides and in particular lauric acid in coconut oil may help to disrupt the viruses' membranes and interfere with their development.

• **Cardio-protective:** Coconut contains the fatty acids caprylic, lauric, myristic, palmitic, stearic, oleic, and linoleic and medium-chain triglycerides which permits these fatty acids to be directly absorbed by the intestine and routed straight to the liver for speedy metabolism and energy production. The medium chain triglycerides in coconut oil do not biosynthesize and transport cholesterol. Also, coconut water contains potassium which has beneficial cardio-protective effects.

• **Electrolytes:** Coconuts are rich in the electrolytes calcium, magnesium, phosphorus, and potassium, which are said to help to lower blood pressure, relax the blood vessels, and lower blood pressure.

• **Hypolipidemic:** Virgin coconut oil may inhibit lipid peroxidation due to its high content of coconut protein and polyphenols. These serve to inhibit low-density lipoprotein oxidation, reverse cholesterol transport, and reduce intestinal absorption of cholesterol.

• **Hepatroprotective:** Coconut oil may protect the liver from fatty infiltration or *necrosis*.

• **Hormone-like effects:** Young coconut water is thought to contain phytoestrogen and other sex hormones that may be used in hormone replacement therapy, to help prevent dementia and in wound healing. Products may vary.

• **Immunostimulatory:** Virgin coconut oil that is enriched with zinc may increase cellular immune function. Coconut protein may increase various levels of immune markers. Both observations may indicate significant immune activity.

Red Bell Pepper Soup

- 2 tablespoons coconut oil (refined)
- 8 large red bell pepper, stemmed, seeded, and quartered
- 1 large onion, thinly sliced
- 3 cloves garlic, minced
- 1 teaspoon black pepper
- 1 teaspoon dried oregano
- 2 tablespoons balsamic vinegar
- 1½ tablespoons fresh thyme, divided

1. Coat 6-quart or larger slow cooker with oil. Add bell peppers, onion, garlic, black pepper and oregano; stir gently to combine. Cover and cook on HIGH 4 hours, or until bell peppers are very tender; stirring halfway through cooking.

2. Purée soup in slow cooker using immersion blender or transfer in batches to blender or food processor and blend until smooth. Stir in balsamic vinegar. Ladle soup into bowls; garnish with thyme.

Makes 4 to 6 servings

This slow cooker recipe, Red Bell Pepper Soup, is a beautiful red-orange color, made with coconut oil, red bell peppers, onion, garlic, oregano, balsamic vinegar and fresh thyme. Red bell peppers are rich in antioxidant vitamins A and C and of course coconut oil lends some additional antioxidants and lusciousness. The balsamic vinegar adds piquancy.

Antibacterial and Antiviral Properties

These are how some of these theoretical medicinal effects of coconuts translate into practical usages. As always, check with a health care practitioner before starting any of these practices.

Acne

Coconut oil with its antibacterial properties from lauric acid may be applied to skin that is broken out or has acne. Use a clean cotton ball that is soaked with warm coconut oil and apply it first to a small area of the face or body to observe if there are any reactions. Then another clean cotton ball filled with warmed coconut oil can be swabbed over the face and body. The lauric acid may inhibit bacterial growth and reduce inflammation. A naturally scented essential oil, such as lemon or rosemary may be added, if desired. This application should be repeated as needed. It may eventually reduce blotches, redness and/or irritation.

To keep the scalp and hair smelling fresh and clean, a few drops of essential oil of choice may be added to the warmed coconut oil before application.

Simple cuts, burns, or other skin injuries may also benefit by this application. The healing properties are again due, in part, to the lauric acid in coconut oil.

Dandruff Remedy

Dandruff may be more than dry skin on the scalp. Dandruff may be produced by an overly oily scalp that causes skin cells to clump together and resemble white flakes; skin conditions that include eczema, psoriasis or *seborrheic dermatitis* (a red, itchy rash that is common in children); or by a fungus that similar to the fungus that causes yeast infections.

Coconut oil may have antifungal properties. When it is rubbed into the scalp it may help old skin cells to slough away. A simple head massage with warmed coconut oil may help to loosen the oily cells that built up, promote healthier oil production and distribution, and improve circulation, which are all good measures to reduce dandruff.

Use the fingertips instead of fingernails to avoid damaging the scalp and increasing the infection. Allow the warmed coconut oil to remain some time on the scalp to revitalize it. Covering the scalp and hair with a cap or wrap will enhance the process.

Deodorant

Coconut oil is moisturizing and may help to keep the armpits virtually free from bumps, chafing, flakes, or itching while smelling pleasant. The lauric acid in coconut oil may also be antibacterial and antifungal when coconut oil is used as a deodorant.

A small scoop of coconut oil may be used right from the container and applied to the underarms, face or legs as needed. Any excess should be wiped with a clean, dry cloth. The thin coconut layer should be left to dry before dressing as to avoid any stains on garments.

Coconut Deodorant

¼ cup baking soda

½ cup arrowroot or cornstarch

Essential oil (such as lavender, lemon, rosemary or thyme), if desired

6 tablespoons coconut oil

Sterilized, dry glass jar with lid

1. Blend baking soda and arrowroot or cornstarch in medium-sized bowl.

2. Add a few drops of essential oil, if desired.

3. Add coconut oil; blend with back of spoon until well blended.

4. Store in sterilized glass jar in cool location.

A simpler method is to mix about one tablespoon of arrowroot powder into three to four tablespoons of coconut oil and blend well. A little beeswax can be used to help to solidify the mixture.

Coconut deodorant can be easily made with baking soda and cornstarch, scented or unscented. Coconut oil may help to decrease the bacteria that cause body odor.

Disinfectant

Coconut soap has been shown to be effective as a disinfecting agent when it is used to brush dentures. Lautericide, a disinfectant that contains coconut acid, has bacterial and fungicidal properties.

Sore Throat

When you have a cold, a swish of coconut oil with its inherent lauric acid may be soothing for sore throats and may decrease the length of time of discomfort, improve immunity, and prevent additional sore throats.

Immunological Properties

Let's look at some specific conditions and remedies!

A teaspoon of apple cider vinegar, warm water, and coconut oil may be especially soothing and restorative for sore throats.

Allergens

Allergy sufferers are plagued with a host of allergic symptoms, sometimes yearlong. These may include coughing, headaches, itchy eyes, sinusitis, sneezing, or respiratory infections. Due to the reported antibacterial, antimicrobial, and antiviral properties of coconut oil, it has been said to help decrease sensitivities to allergens in the environment and allergic conditions, including respiratory discomfort, sinus pressure, and sneezing.

One to three tablespoons daily of coconut oil in food or on its own may help to protect the body against common allergic ailments and/or diminish their severity. A little coconut oil that is lightly swabbed at the base of the nostrils may also be effective. Thanks to the lauric acid in coconut oil, the body may then be able to build up its defense.

Bumps and Bruises

A few tablespoons of coconut oil with its anti-inflammatory properties taken daily reportedly may help the body to efficiently and quickly repair, rebuild, and restore.

Bruising occurs when there is trauma to the skin and broken blood vessels manifest in colors that range from green to blackish-purple. The lauric acid and medium-chain triglycerides in coconut oil are anti-inflammatory and preventative against future injuries to the body.

After a minor bruise, ice the injured area first. Ice compresses and alleviates the swelling and pain. Ice may also help decrease the enlargement of the bruise, while it speeds up the healing process. Ice should be placed on the bruised region for about 15 to 20 minutes and repeated as needed.

Then the bruised area should be elevated to help prevent the accumulation of blood, discoloration and swelling. Gently massaging the bruised area helps to break down the injured blood cells and improves circulation and the lymphatic process that removes toxins, waste, and other unwanted body materials.

One to three tablespoons of coconut oil can then be applied to the injured area with a clean, dry cotton ball. Then a gentle massage with clean fingertips may help to distribute the remnants of the broken blood vessels so that they may dissipate and be internally removed.

Some preventative measures may also help those with allergies such as showering after periods of being outdoors during high allergy seasons; driving with the car windows shut; and/or consuming local honey to build immunity against the local allergens.

Older adults tend to bruise more easily than when they were younger because the skin becomes less flexible, thinner and has less fat for cushioning. Women tend to bruise more easily than men. The tendency to bruise easily may be genetic.

As a component of salve, coconut oil may nourish the skin and transfer essential oils and herbs, depending upon the salve's composition. With its antibacterial and antioxidant properties, the coconut oil within the salve may also help to protect and heal the body.

Add dried herbs to coconut oil, and blend in beeswax and essential oils of choice for a soothing, pleasantly smelling salve for relaxation, rough skin, or sore muscles.

Coconut Oil Salve

- 2 to 3 cups coconut oil
- 8 to 10 ounces dried herbs (such as calendula, comfrey, rosemary or yarrow)
- 1 ounce beeswax per 8 ounces herbal oil

Essential oil (such as lavender, lemon, Roman chamomile or tea tree)

1. Add coconut oil to upper pot of a double boiler.

2. Sprinkle dried herbs over coconut oil.

3. Add water to bottom pot of double boiler; heat to just before simmer.

4. Place pot of coconut oil/herb mixture over pot of heated water; heat until mixture melts, is unified in color, and the herbs are no longer dry.

5. Remove from heat and cool.

6. Drain coconut oil from herbs by slowly pouring through a cheesecloth-lined strainer into medium bowl.

7. Repeat with any remaining oil and herbs if needed.

8. Carefully wring contents of cooled cheesecloth and herbs into bowl until no longer residue.

9. Dispose of any remaining dried herbs and cheesecloth.

10. Add one-ounce beeswax per eight-ounces herb-infused oil back into upper pot of double boiler. Reheat water in lower pot of double boiler just before simmer.

11. Upon melting, add a few drops of essential oils to mixture*. Mix well; set aside to fully cool.

12. Once cooled, pour the herbal mixture into clean, sanitized containers.

*Depending on the essential oil and its freshness, this might require about 10 or more drops of essential oil per one cup of herbal oil. The essential oil can be used on its own or mixed with a complimentary type.

NOTE: The herbal coconut oil salve will semi-harden as coconut oil does. To prevent rancidity, store in refrigerator and remove only enough to use as needed. Warm a tablespoon or more in the palm of the hands as desired.

Fungal Infections

Another reported immunological use of coconut oil is in the prevention of fungal infections. With its antifungal and probiotic attributes, coconut oil may help to rid the body of yeast infections that are caused by the yeast *candida* and its overgrowth. When a cell's mucosal barriers is impeded or the immune system is compromised then candida may invade and trigger infection.

The lauric acid in coconuts may help to reduce the pain and itching that are associated with yeast infections, minimize the spread of yeast infections, and ease the inflammation. A few tablespoons of coconut oil that are ingested daily might be preventative. It is best to check with a health care practitioner before using coconut oil topically.

Insect Repellent

The use of *dodecanoic acid* (DDA) against ticks has been validated and DDA is patented. The active ingredient DDA is a naturally occurring *carboxylic acid*, which is the broader classification of the acids that are found in coconut oil. Coconut oil has also been shown to show some repellency against mosquitos.

Lice Prevention and Treatment

Lice are wingless insects that live externally on warm-blooded hosts that include every species of bird and mammal. In number, lice are called *louse* and their eggs are called *nits* that hatch into *nymphs*.

Lice favor clean hair and scalp so that they can freely move throughout the hair and their nits can create strong bonds to the hair strands. Lice are contagious, irritating, and are often difficult to remove; however, lice generally do not spread disease. If the scalp is scratched and then inflamed, infection may develop.

Lice can only live off of the human scalp a short amount of time since their only food source is human blood. They cannot live on any other species but they can reside on bed linens, carpets, and furniture—that's why it is important to do a thorough cleaning after lice infestation.

Dogs and other animals have a form of lice that is uniquely theirs. This form cannot survive on humans.

Over-the-counter (OTC) products with highly concentrated pesticides may be absorbed through the skin. Also, head lice may build up resistance to them and these OTC products may become ineffective at killing nits.

Instead, different types of oils have been used around the world for centuries to treat lice. While coconut oil may not kill lice, it may temporarily immobilize and suffocate them. The viscous consistency of coconut oil is sometimes effective in killing adult lice, but it may be ineffective in killing nits or baby louse. In order for the nits to die they must be manually removed from the strands of hair where they have infiltrated.

A natural treatment for lice infestation is as follows:

• Rinse the scalp with apple vinegar

• Let the apple cider vinegar remain on the hair to dry.

• Carefully comb the hair while removing as many nits as possible.

• Mix a combination of one cup of coconut oil and 1 to 3 tablespoons of essential oils (such as anise or ylang-ylang with their antibacterial, antifungal and insecticidal properties)

• Apply this mixture to the hair and scalp.

• Cover the hair and scalp with a thin shower cap or wrap and allow it to set for 12 or more hours, if possible.

• The hair should then be shampooed, rinsed and combed with a special lice comb that has small, closely spaced teeth to remove as many nits and eggs as are visible.

• This process can be repeated until the lice are eliminated.

Massage Oil

The type of massage oil that one chooses may either enliven or soothe the body depending upon its consistency and aroma. Coconut oil provides lubrication and moisturizing for kneading, rubbing, and relaxing the body.

Simply blend one cup of coconut oil with a few drops of essential oils of choice, such as sweet and fragrant orange, geranium, rose, vanilla or ylang-ylang, or spicy and invigorating bergamot, cypress, fennel, frankincense, helichrysum, lavender, myrrh, lemon grass, or rosemary. The sweeter essential oils may promote relaxation while the spicier oils may be uplifting. Essential oils are concentrated and work best when they are blended into a nourishing medium, such as coconut oil with its wonderful skin-friendly and protective capric and lauric acids.

Nose Bleed Prevention

Coconut oil may be used to prevent nosebleeds that are attributed to dry nostrils from air pollutants, allergies, or extremes in temperature or humidity. These conditions often result in inflammation or cracks in the mucus membranes and subsequent bleeding.

A little coconut oil that is dabbed onto the base of the nostrils may help to soften them and prevent cracking or drying. Make sure that the hands are clean, especially under the fingernails. Coconut oil taken by mouth may also help to keep these tissues pliable from the inside by protecting and strengthening the capillaries of the nasal passages. Make sure that your antioxidant intake especially vitamins A and C) is also sufficient.

Soothes Bee Stings, Bug Bites, Minimal Scrapes and Scratches

The three ways that coconut oil affects simple wound healing are:

1. That it has the ability to accelerate *re-epithelialization* (the process of covering a wound's surface),

2. It improves antioxidant enzyme activity

3. It stimulates higher collagen cross-linking within the tissue being repaired to form a barrier between the skin and the environment.

Bugs can transmit microbes and foster disease and illness, especially when the skin is infected. Coconut oil with capric and lauric acids combined with tea tree oil (a natural derivative of the *melaleuca* plant) is an easy, effective, and reportedly safe solution for bites.

Simply add about 10 drops of tea tree oil to about one-half cup of warmed coconut oil and blend well. This mixture can be applied with a clean cotton ball to the skin, or poured into a clean spray bottle so that a thin layer can be sprayed over the affected areas. This mixture may help to soothe the skin, safeguard the skin against future insect bites, and moisturize the skin in the process.

Sun Protection

Consuming coconuts and applying coconut oil to the skin may help to protect the skin from the sun both from the inside and outside of the body. Damaging UVA and UVB rays may lead to skin cancer or other skin disorders besides drying and weathering the skin that exacerbates aging skin. UVA rays may penetrate deep within the thickest layer of the skin, or the dermis. UVB rays may often burn the superficial layers of the skin and may play a key role in skin cancer.

Coconut oil alone or blended with equal amounts of cocoa butter may help to soften dehydrated, sun-dried skin, and retard peeling from sunburn. It may not be effective against the harsh effects of the sun with a Sun Protection Factor (SPF) of 4 or less depending upon laboratory testing, especially if homemade.

Coconut oil may help heal small nicks from shaving on the face, as well as on the underarms and legs.

Replacements of Fluid and Electrolytes

Coconut water is low in calories (about 5.45 calories per ounce or abut 65.4 calories per 12-ounces depending upon the brand) and naturally fat- and cholesterol free. Coconut water contains more potassium than one medium banana (862 milligrams per 12-ounces of coconut water versus 422 milligrams in one medium banana). Benefits like these are why coconut water is often called "Mother Nature's Sports Drink."

Coconut water is naturally refreshing with its sweet and nutty taste. Its natural sugar content is easily digestible and it contains some electrolytes that are needed for rehydration, specifically potassium and sodium. Coconut water also contains calcium and minor amounts of magnesium, phosphorus, and zinc.

Ounce for ounce, when typical coconut water is compared to common sports drinks it can be seen that coconut water is slightly less caloric per ounce, with slightly less sugar, more potassium, and less sodium. The reason why some sports drinks are so effective for rehydration is that their composition of nutrients closely resembles that of perspiration. This feature may increase their effectiveness and appeal.

Coconut Water	Sports Drinks
5.45 calories/ounce	6.25 calories/ounce
1.3 grams sugar	1.75 grams sugar
61 milligrams potassium	3.75 milligrams potassium
5.45 milligrams sodium	13.75 milligrams sodium

Coconut water contains less sugar than some sodas and fruit juices, but its sugars may add up if coconut water is consumed in excess.

Still, some athletes feel that coconut water is very hydrating because it is not overly sweet and coconut water is so drinkable. A study of professional athletes has shown that coconut water (especially when it was enhanced with sodium) replenishes body fluids similarly to sports drinks and water as long as it is flavored and athletes tolerate significant amounts to keep hydrated. For rehydration, coconut water has been shown to be as good as sports drinks and causes less fullness, nausea, and stomach upset when it is consumed in large amounts that are required for rehydration.

Since hydration is critical for everyone, but particularly for recreational and professional athletes, if the taste and hydrating abilities of coconut water encourage people to consume more fluids, then coconut water may be considered an effective hydrating beverage.

Since people need to be hydrated daily, the natural hydrating capacity of coconut water with its potassium supply is beneficial. Keep in mind that fruits, vegetables, and dairy products are also ample in potassium and should be part of a well-rounded diet.

If people lose weight after heavy exercise and/or perspire heavily, then neither coconut water nor sports drinks may provide enough replacement carbohydrates or sodium. Their diet may need extra calorie and sodium supplementation post exercise. A handful of pretzels or raisins will supply some simple and complex carbohydrates for immediate and longer energy and the sodium in the pretzels will to help to replenish this electrolyte.

Making Your Own

In this hectic world in which we live, it might be overwhelming to considering making some of these home-made products and potential remedies compared to the ease of purchasing their commercial varieties.

This may be true; however, coconut-based products may be more economical, environmental friendly, and in some cases, work as effectively if not better than their commercial counterparts.

It might be fun to try an easy mixture and notice any results. The coconut just may find its place as a go-to ingredient for many surprising invaders that cause harm.

Green Coconut Water Smoothie

½   cup frozen banana, cut into chunks

¼   cup frozen mango, cut into chunks

2   cups fresh greens (kale, spinach, watercress or mixed greens)*

1   cup coconut water (plus more to thin)

1   teaspoon ground walnuts or pistachios, to garnish (optional)

1. Combine the first four ingredients into a blender.

2. Blend until smooth, frothy consistency.

3. Thin with additional coconut water, if desired.

4. Garnish with ground walnuts or pistachios, if desired.

Makes about 3 to 3¾ cups, depending upon how greens are packed into cup measure.

Coconut the Beautiful

Not only can people consume the goodness of the coconut, people can *wear* coconuts, too—on their face and body, that is! Coconuts have been extolled for their radiant properties in beauty and personal care. Coconut oil may be one of the best skin creams, hydrating serums, and moisturizing lotions available. That said, some of the magic-like qualities of coconuts are valid while others maybe more folklore. Let's explore!

The unique properties of coconuts make them extremely versatile and useful for a myriad of beauty and hygienic habits. This chapter will sort out the rights and wrongs for using coconuts for beautification purposes.

> Homemade coconut lip balm can be made clear or colored, almost fragrant-free, or scented.

Skin Care

The cell membranes in the skin are made up of three fat-containing substances: *glycolipids* (lipids with a carbohydrate component that helps to identify cells), *phospholipids* (lipids with a phosphate component that provide structure and function to cells), and cholesterol (the waxy, fat-like substance that is found in all cells of the body).

Phospholipids, made of saturated and unsaturated fatty acids, are the largest component of cell membranes. The balance of these three fatty acids is important for proper cell function and it is critical to human and animal health. The fatty acids in coconuts contribute to a healthy balance of these fatty acids in the cell membranes of the skin.

Aging, heat and cold, medications, skin treatments, and the sun can affect the hydration of the skin in a multitude of ways. Replacing this hydration can be done both externally and internally.

Coconut lip balm

- 2 ounces coconut oil
- 2 ounce clean, sterilized, dry container

Microwavable bowl

Clean spoon for mixing

Additional flavored or non-flavored oil, if desired (argan, avocado, jojoba or olive)

Lipstick, if desired

1. Place coconut oil and a few drops of additional flavored or non-flavored oil (if desired) into microwavable bowl.

2. Mix well with spoon until smooth consistency.

3. Add a few shavings from lipstick tube, if desired.

4. Microwave about 10 to 30 seconds depending upon microwave setting until mixture melts.

5. Remove from microwave; blend again with spoon.

6. When cool, place in refrigerator to harden.

7. Keep cool; warm with fingertip to apply.

Proper hydration is essential for the skin's cell membranes. The surface skin cells do not dry out as fast or as much and the dead skin cells are reduced or are easily eliminated. As a result, the skin's pores do not get as clogged with dirt and impurities and excess oils do not accumulate, which also reduces the possibility of acne and infections. Firmness and natural elasticity are generally retained and stretch marks and wrinkling also may be reduced in appearance.

Coconut oil provides hydration and essential fatty acids for healthy skin along with proper skin care. Coconut oil helps to protect the skin from free radicals and their aging effects and may help to improve the skin's appearance with its anti-aging benefits. Coconut oil acts as an antioxidant since it is stable, resists oxidation, and contributes some vitamin E, an antioxidant vitamin.

When coconut oil is absorbed into the skin and connective tissues, it may help to reduce the appearance of fine lines and wrinkles. It accomplishes this by supporting the strength and suppleness of connective tissues. It also aids in the exfoliation of the outer layer of dead skin cells, which makes the skin look smoother. Plus, it has a delightful aroma that bathes the skin to the enjoyment of the wearer and those in the immediate vicinity, so no other cologne or perfume may be necessary for use.

Skin-enhancing Qualities of Coconut Oil

Several of the skin-enhancing qualities of coconut oil and coconut products include:

Acne relief: Coconut oil helps to keep skin hydrated and the pores open to reduce impurities and acne-related skin conditions.

Age spot minimizer: Coconut oil may diminish the look of age spots when used on a regular basis. It may accomplish this by keeping the area of the age spots and also the skin around the age spots supple.

Anti-aging defense: By smoothing the look of wrinkled skin, coconut oil may help to make skin appear younger. Younger skin does have more moisture that may dissipate over the years.

Baby lotion/massage oil: Warmed coconut oil with essential oil such as lavender, mint, rosemary or vanilla help to provide a relaxing, rejuvenating massage.

Bath/body moisturizer: Scented (or unscented) coconut massage oil can be applied to the skin both in and out of the bath or shower.

Body balm: Coconut-oil-based body balm is dense, hydrates, and repairs. It is similar to a lotion with light consistency that moistures but does not repair and a cream that is usually thicker, but is formulated for the face.

Body scrub: Coconut oil and coarse salt or sugar acts as an exfoliator for dry skin. Either fragrant (such a eucalyptus or lavender) or non-fragrant essential oils may be added.

Coconut body scrub

¼ to ½ **cup granulated sugar or coarse salt**

½ **cup coconut oil**

Essential oil (citrus or herbal, such as lemon or rosemary), optional

1. Combine granulated sugar, coarse salt or combination of sugar and salt with coconut oil. Do not heat to melt the coconut oil.

2. Add a few drops of essential oil if desired; blend ingredients well.

3. Place into sanitized, dry container.

Coconut body scrub acts as an all-in-one body wash, exfoliator and moisturizer. It can be made with granulated sugar, salt or a combination of these two ingredients and with or without essential oil.

Bruise reducer: Coconut oil may not directly reduce the appearance of bruises, but similar to its effects on scars, sores, and stretch marks, it may promote the healing of the surrounding skin over time.

Cold sore reliever: Cold sores, often due to viruses, may benefit from coconut oil's anti-viral properties due to its composition of lauric and stearic fatty acids, know for their curative properties.

Deodorant: Coconut oil mixed with arrowroot powder, baking soda, cornstarch and scented or unscented essential oils can be used as a natural deodorant.

Diaper rash relief: Unless there is a known sensitivity to coconuts, a thin layer of coconut oil may provide some relief for chafed skin.

Dry feet remedy: Apply coconut oil to cracked skin and dry spots to smooth dry feet, especially in winter or after hot, dry summer sun.

Emollient: An emollient is a cream or an ointment that acts like a moisturizer. It is designed to help make the *epidermis* (outer layer of the skin) softer and suppler. Versatile coconut oil can be used as a base for homemade bath or body emollients or moisturizers.

Facial mask: The antioxidants and fatty acids in coconut oil help to lubricate, smooth, and soften the skin when it is mixed with baking soda, lemon, turmeric, or yogurt as a facial mask.

Lip balm: Coconut oil is a remedy for chapped lips since it is semisolid at room temperature and can easily be spread by fingertips. Coconut balm is particularly soothing for the lips. A touch of natural extract, such as vanilla gives coconut lip balm a tropical flavor.

Makeup Remover: Apply coconut oil directly to the face to cleanse it, or let it remain on the skin to rehydrate. Be particularly careful around the eyes so as not to over-oil them.

Night cream: Apply coconut oil at night for its maximum moisturizing benefits, particularly around fine lines or wrinkles. A little left on the pillow at night will also moisturize the hair.

Nursing mothers' aid/nipple soother: Use coconut oil delicately around sore or cracked nipples to rehydrate, soften, and heal. This practice can be checked with an obstetrician or nurse midwife first before trying.

Shave cream: Coconut oil helps to provide a smoother, closer shave that leaves the arms, face and legs evenly soft and moisturized.

Skin protection (dishpan hands, eczema, psoriasis): Coconut oil and coconut balm offers relief from allergic and chronic skin conditions that can be heightened by over-exposure to chemicals, sun, water and other skin-damaging factors. Check with an allergist first before applying to very sensitive skin.

Stretch mark/scar reducer: Pregnant women and people with minor scrapes and scratches can use coconut oil as a topical treatment for marks and scars. Coconut oil probably will not directly cause fading, but it may help to prevent dark spots and/or blisters from forming. Coconut oil may also help the surrounding skin retain its moisture and healthy glow.

Sun block/soother: Coconut oil is soothing and has a natural sunscreen of SPF 4. It is still sensible to stay out of the direct contact of the sun. Sunscreens with a higher SPF should offer more protection from the sun's harmful ultraviolet (UV) radiation.

Under-eye cream: Applied under the eyes and around fine lines, coconut oil combats a dried-out appearance and it is light and delicate for most skin types.

To make a simple, soothing shave cream, use a combination of ⅔ cup coconut oil, ⅔ cup shea nut oil or shea butter and ¼ cup olive oil or grapeseed oil, blended with the following optional ingredients: a few drops of essential oils, 2 tablespoons of baking soda and the contents of two vitamin E capsules, beaten until frosting consistency.

Hair and Nails

Like healthy skin, healthy hair and nails are formed, to a great part, by a healthy diet that includes proper hydration. An unhealthy diet can lead to hair that is brittle, dull, or lifeless; a scalp that is flaky; nails that break and chip easily; and ragged cuticles. Coconut oil plays a role in radiant hair, smooth nails, and neat cuticles due to its fat content and along with coconut milk and coconut water helps hydration.

Coconut oil can be applied directly to the scalp, hair, nails, and nail beds. While excess coconut oil can be removed, the residue can remain for a healthy glow and moisturizing. Or, coconut oil can be mixed with some warm water, gently applied to the scalp, then allowed to soak into the scalp and hair before washing with shampoo and conditioner—coconut-based, of course! Plus, when coconuts are consumed they help to nourish the hair and nails from the inside out!

These are some of the uses of coconut products to enrich the hair and nails:

Adds shine and conditions hair: Coconut oil hydrates hair over time since it replaces the natural oils that shampoos tend to strip away. As a leave-in conditioner, coconut oil may condition the hair immediately and then benefit the hair over time. Some people think that application to wet hair is more desirable for sealing in moisture than on dry hair, but water and oil do not mix (consider vinegar and oil salad dressing), so it is best to experiment.

Dandruff control: Dandruff along with dry scalp may be chronic problems. The daily use of coconut oil literally confronts the root of the problem. A light head massage with warm coconut oil may also be invigorating.

Defrizzes hair and reduces split ends: Frizzy hair is often the result of dry conditions: too many chemicals in shampoos and conditioners, coloring, perms, or general over-processing. Coconut oil helps to calm frizzy hair and restore its luster. While regular trims are best for split ends, coconut oil may tame their unruliness in the short-term before the haircut.

Enhances eyebrows and eyelashes: Coconut oil may penetrate the hair follicles in the eyebrows and eyelashes and prevent a scaly look so that they appear to be soft and shiny.

Provides protection from ultraviolet (UV) radiation: Sunlight helps to create a pre-cursor of vitamin D on the skin's surface that is necessary for healthy bones and teeth, the heart, and immune function. But too much UV radiation may damage the skin and lead to some cancers. Coconut oil and its richness provide some measures of protection. But the wisest advice is to stay out of dangerous noon-day or tropical sun.

Reduces fungal infections: Coconut oil with its anti-microbial properties may help to prevent fungal infections of the nails (particularly toenails) and scalp. Coconut oil is even said to reduce *candida*, a systemic fungal infection. Make sure to check with a health care practitioner for use of specific advice.

Softens cuticles: Coconut balm or coconut oil soothes rough and ragged cuticles before they get out of hand. When either of these nurturing coconut products is applied to the nail base, they may enhance the nails and hands.

Stimulates nail growth: Nails need a moisturized environment in which to thrive. Coconut oil helps to prevent the nails from becoming too overly brittle and split that may hinder their growth. Ample protein, biotin, B-complex vitamins, calcium, iron, magnesium, omega-3 fatty acids, and zinc are some of the nutrients that are needed for healthy nails.

You can use coconut oil as a cleanser for your hairbrush and comb! Remove any tangled hair from the hairbrushes and combs. Rub warmed coconut oil completely throughout the hairbrushes and combs and let set a few hours. Wash the hairbrushes and combs well and dry with a clean, dry cloth. A little residue may be desirable to revitalize the bristles and teeth, plus it might transfer to the hair the next time they are used.

Supports natural chemical balances in hair and nails: The body is a maze of natural chemicals and reactions that maintain its many functions. On low-fat diets, sometimes there is not enough fat or even protein for normal operations. Coconuts and their products may help support the body's quest for equilibrium of nutrient intake to keep it working smoothly.

Treats hair and scalp: Warmed coconut oil can be applied to the hair and scalp to treat dry hair before using shampoo and conditioner. The longer that it is left on the hair and scalp, the greater its moisturizing benefits. Stronger hair may be spared from dry ends that break or split up the hair and into the hair shaft.

Wards off infection: If used regularly, coconut oil may form a protective barrier on the skin around the nails to impede some common infections. Dry, cracked skin is more vulnerable. Make sure manicures are both safe and sanitary.

Muscles

Proper muscle tone requires a muscle-building and maintenance program. One needs muscle-building exercises, a regular exercise routine, and healthy muscle cells and surrounding tissues that support all of this muscular work. Of course, a good diet with protein and muscle building nutrients such as B-vitamins, calcium, magnesium, and vitamins C, D, and E are vital.

The right kinds of fatty acids in sufficient quantity are essential to build and maintain healthy cellular membranes within muscle cells. Coconuts and coconut oil with their saturated fats supply some of this raw material. The size of muscles depends on genetic predisposition and on a dedicated muscle-building program, but a balanced diet supports these factors.

Cellulite, or subcutaneous fat within fibrous connective tissue, makes the skin look dimpled and nodular. Cellulite is common in the pelvic region, including the abdomen, buttocks and lower limbs. Its causes may be genetic, hormonal, or lifestyle.

Effective treatments for cellulite are varied and debated. The use of coconut oil to reduce the look and texture of cellulite is one of these deliberations. The theory is that the human body requires certain substances to help to metabolize or break down its fat stores into energy.

The medium-chain triglycerides and lauric acid in coconut oil help to reduce inflammation, boost metabolism, and break down fatty accumulations. They work in conjunction with specific enzymes that break down fats into fatty acids and glycerol that are further broken down in the liver or used for energy. The enzymes are activated by the hormones epinephrine, glucagon, and growth hormone.

In the process of using these medium-chain triglycerides and lauric acid the skin may become more elastic, silkier, and smoother in appearance and the bumpy, holey look of cellulite may be diminished.

Spider veins are small and twisted blood vessels that may be visible through the skin. They may look more pronounced when the skin is dry or saggy in appearance. Coconut oil can be gently massaged into the areas where spider veins appear on the face or legs. They may help to restore the surrounding cells and detract from the redness.

Teeth and Gums

The fat-soluble vitamins A, D, E, and K require fat for proper absorption and assimilation. In particular, vitamins A and D are essential for strong bones and teeth. By remineralizing tooth enamel, these vitamins help to build up the protective qualities of the teeth and help to guard against cavities. The anti-inflammatory, analgesic, and antipyretic (fever-reducing) properties of coconut oil may help to defend the teeth against decay. Healthy teeth and gums are one of the body's first lines against infection.

In particular, coconut oil:

• **Helps prevent periodontal disease and tooth decay:** Due to coconut oil's anti-inflammatory abilities, it may help to keep the mouth and gums healthy and even fight infection.

- **Improves calcium and magnesium absorption and supports the development of strong bones and teeth:** Coconut oil with its medium-chain triglycerides may have the capacity to increase calcium and magnesium absorption, which in turn may help to promote strong bones and teeth. Many other dietary factors are still in play, such as calcium, phosphorus, potassium, and vitamin A, C, D, and K intake.

- **Whitens teeth and acts as a mouthwash:** With its antifungal and antibacterial properties, coconut oil that is mixed with a little baking soda makes a natural whitening and protective paste. A few drops of an essential oil, such as anise with its licorice taste or mint or may be added.

- Gargling with a spoonful of coconut oil may help to reduce oral bacteria and contribute to fresher breath and healthier gums. You can learn more about this practice of "oil pulling" in Chapter 9.

Sun Damage and Aging

Sun damage is due to sun exposure throughout the years from everyday activities to conscious sun bathing. The changes in the earth's ozone layer are also responsible for undesirable ultraviolet (UV) radiation. Fair-skinned and darker-skinned individuals are both prone to sun damage; however, fairer-skinned individuals are more at risk.

In some parts of the world where there is intense and non-stop sun exposure, residents do not seem to have the same type of sun damage than they do in other locations. It may be that their local diets are more abundant in antioxidant–rich foods and vegetables that feed and protect the skin from the inside out.

Cellular degeneration may be caused by *free radicals* in the environment. Free radicals may be formed as the result of exposure to sunlight and air pollutants, but they may also be due to alcohol consumption, diet, drugs, exercise, inflammation, smoking, and one's diet.

One method to delay or prevent cellular degeneration from free radicals is with a diet that is rich in antioxidants (substances that help to halt oxidation which causes cellular destruction). Coconut oil has some antioxidants, but it is more valuable for its saturated fatty acids.

A diet that is high in polyunsaturated fatty acids may lead to cellular membrane instability and make one more prone to cellular damage by the sun and environmental factors. Saturated fats are more protective.

Kiwi Green Dream

- ¾ **cup coconut water**
- 2 **kiwis, peeled and quartered**
- ½ **cup frozen pineapple chunks**
- ½ **avocado, pitted and peeled**
- 1 **tablespoon chia seeds**

Combine water, kiwis, pineapple, and avocado in blender; blend until smooth. Add chia seeds; blend until smooth. Serve immediately.

Makes 2 servings

Kiwi Green Dream is a smoothie made with coconut water, kiwis, frozen pineapple, avocado and chia seeds. Its vibrant green color that is speckled with kiwi seeds is inviting and its coconut-pineapple flavor is refreshing and reminiscent of lazy, indulgent beach days.

Coconut oil, when liberally applied to the skin, also helps to retain the skin's moisture and shiny appearance in hot, dry conditions and promotes all-over tanning, if desirable.

Aging affects the skin since it loses hydration and flexibility and the healing process takes longer than in younger skin. When coupled with the constant exposure to ultraviolet radiation and increased damage by free radicals, aging skin may look dry, old, saggy, and wrinkly.

Coconut oil to the rescue! Coconut oil may be used to treat weathered skin or even to help guard against the grim ravages of ultraviolet radiation. However, coconut oil may not be a cure-all for advanced skin problems. Before using, check with a specialist for prescribed care.

Traditional Beauty Rituals

Many diverse cultures worldwide have valued coconuts and specifically coconut oil for centuries for various beauty rituals. This is in additional to their culinary uses and traditional medicinal remedies that may include abscesses, asthma, baldness, bronchitis, bruises, burns, colds, constipation, cough, dropsy, dysentery, earache, fever, flu, gingivitis, gonorrhea, irregular or painful menstruation, jaundice, kidney stones, lice, malnutrition, nausea, rash, scabies, scurvy, skin infections, sore throat, swelling, syphilis, toothache, tuberculosis, tumors, typhoid, ulcers, upset stomach, weakness, wounds, and many more. The use of coconuts and coconut oil for these treatments varies from culture to culture and many of the miraculous claims may have other causations and cures.

Coconuts and coconut products have also been respected for thousands of years for their esteemed importance in local folklore. This reverence for the coconut and its oil helps explain its variety of usages in the following settings:

Central and South America

In the coastal jungles of Central and South America, coconuts and coconut oil are used both as food and as medicine by traditional healers who attempt to nourish and treat the ill back to health, including minor maladies such as skin ailments.

Ethiopia, Nigeria, Somalia

Palm kernel oil, which is an oil that is very similar in scope to coconut oil, is a very popular treatment for a host of illnesses and conditions in these parts of Africa.

India

Coconut oil is an important component of *Ayurvedic medicine*, a type of alternative or complementary form of traditional medicine that was established more than 3,000 years ago in India. Ayurvedic medicine is based on the belief that health and wellness depend on a delicate balance between the mind, body and spirit.

In addition to coconut oil's medicinal applications, Indian women are said to have favored coconut oil to give their hair luster and volume.

Indonesia

In Indonesia women historically applied coconut oil on their hair and body to keep their hair and skin healthy, as well as using it for culinary purposes. Coconut oil is still important for these reasons and for the Indonesian economy today.

Jamaica

Coconut oil was the "go-to" elixir for common illnesses and it was reportedly used as a health tonic since it was considered to be heart healthy. Today, coconut oil is used to bind the natural protein structure of hair, seal the hair after moisturizing, tame frizz, and as a pre-shampoo treatment and scalp massage

Panama

Panamanians have been known to drink a glass of coconut oil as a preventative against illness and to speed recovery. Today, Panamanian coconut oil is found throughout its Pacific beaches, where it is used for healthy skin, hair care, massage oil, make-up removal, weight loss, and for cooking.

Kitava

Kitava is one of the tiny Trobriand Islands of Papua New Guinea. The Kitavan population consumes a significant amount of coconuts and while their lifespan may be shorter than others worldwide, they are healthy and fit—much attributed to their coconut-rich diet. Kitavans are said to possess healthy skin without acne.

Papua New Guinea

The native residents of Papua New Guinea have been using virgin coconut oil for centuries for cooking, treating cuts and bruises, hair treatments, and as a skin moisturizer. Papua New Guinea coconut oil is considered to be one of the best coconut oils in the world due to its pristine and unspoiled remote growing regions. The native residents of Papua New Guinea have used this type of coconut oil on their hair as a convenient and natural hair conditioner and to tame its coarseness.

Philippines

In the Philippines, coconut oil that is rubbed throughout the hair is said to maintain color, shininess, and thickness throughout old age. It is also allegedly used for healing bruises, burns, cuts, and even broken bones. When coconut oil is massaged into aching joints and muscles, it offers relief and comfort according to these islanders.

Samoa

The native healers of Samoa used coconut oil as a natural remedy for different types of illness and injuries. Samoan mothers were reported to have used coconut oil to massage their children's bodies so that they would have healthy skin without blemishes or infections and strong bones. The soft spot on infants' heads was gently massaged with coconut oil as a safeguard and teething babies were massaged with coconut oil to reduce any pain they might feel.

Sri Lanka and Thailand

Coconut oil was the mainstay of Sri Lankan and Thai people for cooking, cosmetics, and medicine. The majority of their diets were composed of coconut "cream" and coconut "milk" and coconuts are still staples today. Virgin coconut oil is a much sought after ingredient in beauty and personal care products today.

Butternut Squash in Coconut Milk

- ⅓ cup sweetened flaked coconut
- 2 teaspoons coconut oil
- ½ small onion, finely chopped
- 2 cloves garlic, minced
- 1 cup unsweetened coconut milk
- ¼ cup packed brown sugar
- 1 tablespoon fish sauce
- ⅛ to ¼ teaspoon red pepper flakes
- 1 butternut squash (about 2 pounds), peeled and cut into large cubes
- 1 tablespoon chopped fresh cilantro

1. Preheat oven to 350°F. Spread coconut in baking pan. 5 to 7 minutes, stirring occasionally, until golden brown. Set aside to cool and crisp.

2. Heat oil in large saucepan over medium-high heat. Add onion and garlic; cook and stir 3 minutes or until tender. Add coconut milk, brown sugar, fish sauce and red pepper flakes; stir until sugar is dissolved.

3. Bring mixture to a boil; add squash. Reduce heat to medium. Cover and simmer 30 minutes or until squash is tender. Transfer squash to serving bowl with slotted spoon.

4. Increase heat to high; boil remaining liquid until thickened, stirring constantly. Pour liquid over squash in bowl. Sprinkle with toasted coconut and chopped cilantro. Garnish, if desired.

Makes 4 to 6 servings

Butternut Squash in Coconut Milk combines flaked coconut, coconut oil, onions, garlic, coconut milk, brown sugar, fish sauce, butternut squash, red pepper flakes, and cilantro for a nutritious and delicious combination of tastes that are utterly indulgent.

Tokel

In Tokel in the South Pacific, Tokelauans consume over 60 percent of their calories from coconuts. They are one of the largest consumers of saturated fat in the world and yet they are in relatively good health with no evidence of heart disease.

Zanzibar

Along with beauty, cooking, and health practices, coconut oil was used for candle making, diesel fuel, and as a fuel for lighting.

It is remarkable that the coconut can be so good for you and so beautifying, too. For hundreds of years, people from around the world have captured and utilized this secret for their appearance, health and well-being—not to mention their taste and culinary satisfaction.

Oil-Pulling: Yea or Nay?

This chapter focuses on the ritual of "oil-pulling," which has been used for thousands of years in some parts of the world, but has recently become more popularized in Western countries, including the U.S. Oil-pulling practitioners swish coconut oil in their mouths for several minutes or up to 20 minutes to kill bacteria, improve gum health, prevent cavities and strengthen teeth.

The American Dental Association (ADA) has cautioned against this practice because it states that oil-pulling has not been studied in depth. Plus, some oil-pulling practitioners report that they have noticed no improvement in their overall mouth health.

Still, some oil-pulling advocates believe that the possible pros for oil-pulling seem to outweigh the potential cons. To fully understand the logic behind oil-pulling, read on.

Overview of Oil-Pulling

Oil-pulling is an ancient Indian therapy that involves swishing about one tablespoon of oil inside of the mouth, permitting it to move about the gums, teeth, and tongue, and then spitting the oil out of the mouth. Supposedly the oil "pulls" bacteria, impurities, and other germs from the oral cavity and rids the body of infection. A variety of oils have been used for oil-pulling throughout its use in history.

The use of coconut oil for oil-pulling has increased in popularity. This is probably due to the potential germ-fighting properties of coconut oil due to the lauric acid in coconut oil that attacks "bad" bacteria while it promotes "good" bacteria.

Traditional Uses

To fully understand the process of oil-pulling, one needs to examine its venerated history. Oil-pulling as a type of oral therapy has been practiced in Ayurvedic medicine, one of the oldest systems of medicine in the world, for 3,000 years. Today, many practitioners of Ayurvedic medicine reside in India or Southeast Asia. Ayurvedic medicine may be used singularly as the primary medical approach or in combination with different therapies of conventional Western medicine.

Ayurvedic Medicine

Ayurvedic medicine is a traditional eastern Indian approach to life science that emphasizes balance, harmony, and interconnected-ness. According to Ayurvedic medicine, good health is a balance among body, mind, the senses, and the soul–not the absence of illness.

In fact, the term "Ayurveda" blends the Sanskrit words *ayur* (life) and *veda* (knowledge or science). The key concepts of Ayurvedic medicine are the body's constitution, life forces and universal connectedness. These concepts blend *prakriti* (the body's constitution) with people, their health and the universe (interconnectedness) with *dosha* (life forces) in a not-so dissimilar way to the Greek Biological Humors System of ancient times.

Ayurvedic Medicine and Individualized Health

Ayurvedic medicine does not promote generalized treatments; rather, its premise is individualized, based upon the dominant dosha, or life force of the body and nature. Ayurvedic physicians promote balance. Individualized prescribed treatments may include some combination of diet, exercise, lifestyle recommendations, and unique blends of herbs and of other proprietary ingredients.

These proprietary Ayurvedic products may either be all herbal or made from a combination of herbs, metals, minerals, and other ingredients. The process in which this composition is created is called *rasa shastra*.

Rasa shastra combines metals such as copper, gold, iron, lead, silver, tin, or zinc and other substances that may include coral, feathers, salts, and/or seashells in a purification process that is then combined with herbs to treat various illnesses. A criticism of rasa shastra is that some of these ingredients, such as the heavy metals, may be harmful with improper use or without adequate instruction by a trained Ayurvedic practitioner.

Aside from rasa shastra, another practice in traditional Ayurvedic medicine is the process of gargling to treat different bodily imbalances among the doshas, or life forces. These treatments, called *gandusha* or *kavala graha*, are considered as remedies. They are used to help "cure" such conditions as asthma, diabetes, migraines, and sinusitis as well as for dental and oral care. In *gandusha* one's mouth is filled completely with oil and it is held for about three to five minutes. In *kavala graha* a smaller amount of oil is used, then swished between the teeth and even gargled at the back of the throat.

Ayurvedic Medicine and Oil-Pulling

Historically, in Ayurvedic text, the use of sesame oil is recommended as a preventative to reduce *vata dosha*, or the dryness of the mouth along with burning sensation and inflammation. Coconut oil, herbal oils, and sunflower oil are also recommended, especially after specific ailments are diagnosed. The concept is that by extracting bacteria fungi and toxins from the oral cavity before they move into the body and integrated with the body systems, oil-pulling will both restore and maintain the body's natural balance.

In the ancient Greek Biological Humors System the four "humors" are the metabolic agents of the four elements of the human body. These four humors include blood that represents air, phlegm that represents water, yellow bile that represents fire, and black bile that represents earth. According to this system, to maintain health it is essential to have the right balance of these humors and to ensure their purity. It is natural that organic extra-virgin olive oil-pulling is common today— perhaps a nod to olive oil's Mediterranean roots.

The Physiology of the Mouth and Oil-Pulling

The mouth is a receptacle of both bad and good bacteria. The process of swishing fluids around the oral cavity may dislodge bits and pieces of food and coat the teeth and gums. Oil-pulling may not necessarily "pull" out impurities; rather, it may help to extricate them. Also, oil-pulling should not replace everyday oral hygiene, but it may be an adjunct to daily brushing and flossing. In developing countries where there is not access to modern dental care, oil-pulling may be one of the only alternatives.

Oil-Pulling Benefits

Oil-pulling is said to help fight gingivitis, plaque, and microorganisms that contribute to bad breath. The idea is that the oral microorganisms are encased within a lipid or fatty membrane that adheres to other fats. When oils are swished around the mouth they stick to the undesirable microorganisms within the oral cavity and are spit out after a few minutes of swishing.

Oil-Pulling Practices

The practice of oil-pulling with coconut oil is said to benefit from its lauric acid content with its antimicrobial benefits.

Merely five minutes daily of gentle pushing, sucking, and swishing of coconut oil around the mouth and through the teeth is said to be effective. Smaller amounts are advised (maybe one to two teaspoons to start). As much as twenty minutes daily may be difficult on the jaws. Extended periods of time swishing may pose a risk of *lipoid pneumonia* from accidentally breathing in small amounts of oil.

As the oil mixes with saliva it might become thicker and milkier in appearance. Swallowing is not recommended. A bowl or pot close by for removal is preferred to the sink or toilet. After spitting, it is advised that one rinses well with water. Some people add a little salt to the rinse water. Then brushing and flossing are generally advised afterward.

Oil-Pulling Support

Some small pilot studies have suggested that daily oil swishing may indeed affect oral bacteria. In a 2008 study by Asokan *et al.* that was published in the *Journal of Indian Society of Pedodontics and Preventive Dentistry* it was determined that there was a reduction in *Streptococcus mutans* in the saliva and plaque of adolescents who used oil-pulling with sesame oil in comparison with *chlorhexidine* mouthwash. *Streptococcus mutans* are bacterium that are commonly found in the human oral cavity and significantly contribute to tooth decay. Chlorhexidine mouthwash has antibacterial properties that may control and kill oral bacteria help to prevent tooth decay. This study concluded that oil-pulling may be used as an effective preventative treatment for the maintenance and improvement of oral health.

Another study in 2011 by Asokan *et al.* that was published in the same journal evaluated the effect of oil-pulling with sesame oil on halitosis and the contributing microorganisms, also compared with chlorhexidine mouthwash. Halitosis, considered as "bad breath," may be caused by bacteria that are present below the gum line and the back of the tongue. Disorders of the esophagus, lungs, nasal cavities, stomach, and/or throat may also be contributory.

This study also used adolescents as the study subjects. The researchers concluded that oil-pulling therapy was equally effective to chlorhexidine mouthwash for treating halitosis and the microorganisms that are associated with halitosis.

Asokan postulated that *saponification* (the process by which a vegetable oil or animal fat is mixed with a strong alkali) and *emulsification* (the breakdown of fat globules into tiny droplets) with their mechanical cleansing actions might be indicative of how oil-pulling works. It seems that rinsing with oil leaves an oil residue for these reasons and that swishing or pulling with oil may have a mechanical cleaning action.

In another small pilot study reported by Huributt in 2014 that involved healthy young adults with high levels of oral bacteria, it was concluded that those who used sesame oil to oil-pull experienced a five-fold decrease in oral bacteria compared to a water-only group. Those who used coconut oil to oil-pull experienced a two-fold decrease. When oil-pulling was stopped, the bacteria levels increased. Furthermore, Huributt recommended if people wanted to add oil-pulling to their dental hygiene practice that they should be cautious of allergies or hypersensitivities, use organic, edible oil, and not swallow it.

Oil-Pulling Concern

As stated, the American Dental Association has cautioned again the practice of oil-pulling since it is not studied in depth. Furthermore, the studies previously reported were conducted with eastern Indian subject participants in small sample sizes, and there have not been repeated studies with wider applications.

While the kidneys and the liver serve to remove toxins from the body, the oral cavity is only thought to do so through the practice of Aryuvedic medicine. With more supportable research, exact recommendations for usage, and cautions for any possible side effects, oil-pulling (especially with coconut oil and its antimicrobial lauric acid) may finally see its day.

Oral Health Uses of Coconut Oil

The antibacterial and antifungal properties of coconut oil might be useful to clean dentures, invisible braces, mouth guards, or retainers. Simply rub a little coconut oil on a clean cotton ball and on to the mouth device after rinsing it at night. The lauric acid in the coconut oil may help to keep in clean and reduce bacteria overnight until its next use. Plus, the pleasing smell and taste of coconut oil may be soothing when these mouth devices are used again.

Vitamin E oil with its antioxidant properties may also be used in this manner. Any residue may be absorbed and support healthy gum tissue. Vitamin E oil may be mixed with coconut oil for combined benefits.

As with any therapeutic use of coconut oil, vitamin E oil or any oil for that matter, it is best to check with a dental professional before their use in these and other capacities.

Glazed Parsnips and Carrots

1 **pound parsnips (2 large or 3 medium), quartered lengthwise and cut into sticks**

1 **package (8 ounces) baby carrots**

2 **tablespoons coconut oil (divided)**

Salt and black pepper

¼ **cup orange juice**

1 **tablespoon honey**

⅛ **teaspoon ground ginger**

1. Preheat oven to 425°F.

2. Spread vegetables in shallow roasting pan. Drizzle with 1 tablespoon oil and season with salt and pepper; toss to coat. Bake 30 to 35 minutes or until fork-tender.

3. Combine orange juice, remaining oil, honey and ginger in large skillet. Add vegetables; cook and stir over high heat 1 to 2 minutes or until glazed.

Makes 6 servings

Nutrients for Oral Health

B vitamins (for epithelial cell turnover): Since there are many B-vitamins, each with specific sources, by consuming a wide-range of food and beverages many of the B-vitamin daily requirements should be met.

Parsnips, carrots and orange juice (with antioxidant vitamins A and C), coconut oil, honey and butter combine to make a slightly thickened sweet-tart glazed vegetable side dish that is colorful, crispy, and earthy in its deliciousness.

Calcium-rich foods (for protection and reconstruction of tooth enamel for healthy tooth structure and enhanced enamel mineralization): Food and beverage sources of calcium include almonds, canned salmon, dairy products, dark leafy green vegetables, and fortified soy foods and beverages (including tofu). Raw, shredded coconut meat contains about 11.2 milligrams of calcium per cup.

Folate (for healthy mucosal/connective tissue development and immune function and protection against periodontal disease): Food sources of folate include asparagus, chickpeas, broccoli, Brussels sprouts, fortified breakfast cereals, liver, peas, and spinach. Raw, shredded coconut meat contains about 20.8 micrograms of folate per cup.

Iron (for healthy mucosal/ connective tissues and immune function): Food sources of iron include dark green leafy vegetables such as kale and spinach, iron-fortified breads and breakfast cereals, dried fruit as apricots and raisins, legumes, peas, pork, poultry, red meat, and seafood. Raw, shredded coconut meat contains about 1.9 milligrams of iron per cup.

Omega-3 fatty acids (for healthy mucosal/connective tissues and immune function and inflammatory response modulation): Food sources of omega-3 fatty acids include chia seeds, fatty fish, fish oil, fish roe, seafood, spinach, soybeans, and walnuts.

Phosphorus (for protection and reconstruction of tooth enamel for healthy tooth structure): Food and beverages sources of phosphorus include dairy products, eggs, fish and lean meats. Raw, shredded coconut meat contains about 90.4 milligrams of phosphorus per cup.

Proteins (for healthy tooth structure, musosal/connective tissue development and immune function): Food sources of proteins include both animal and vegetable foods and beverages such as meats, dairy products, grains, legumes and vegetables.

Vitamin A (for healthy mucosal/connective tissue development and immune function): Food sources of vitamin A include bell peppers, cantaloupe, carrots, dark leafy green vegetables, dried apricots, fish, liver, mango, papaya, sweet potatoes, and winter squash.

Vitamin C (for healthy gums and quick would healing): Food sources of vitamin C include broccoli, citrus fruits, peppers, potatoes, spinach, and tomatoes. Raw, shredded coconut meat contains about 2.6 milligrams of vitamin C per cup.

Vitamin D (for healthy mucosal/connective tissue development and immune function and enhanced enamel remineralization): Food and beverage sources of vitamin D include beef liver, cheese, egg yolks, fatty fish such as herring, mackerel, salmon, sardines, and tuna and fortified dairy products.

Zinc (for healthy musosal/connective tissue development and immune function). Food sources of zinc include beef, dairy products, fortified breakfast cereals, legumes, nuts, oysters, seafood (particularly crab and lobster), and whole grains. Raw, shredded coconut meat contains about 0.9 milligrams of zinc per cup.

Salmon and Wild Rice Chowder

- 1 teaspoon coconut oil
- 1 red onion, chopped
- 1 red bell pepper, chopped
- 1 cup green beans, cut into 1-inch pieces
- 1½ teaspoons minced fresh dill weed
- 1 teaspoon salt
- ⅛ teaspoon black pepper
- 3 cups vegetable broth
- 1 cup cooked wild rice
- 12 ounces skinless salmon fillet, cut into 1-inch pieces
- ½ cup milk
- 2 teaspoons all-purpose flour

1. Melt coconut oil in large saucepan over high heat. Add onion, bell pepper and green beans; cook and stir 5 minutes. Stir in dill, salt and black pepper. Pour in broth; bring to a simmer.

2. Add wild rice and salmon to saucepan. Reduce heat to low; cover and simmer 6 to 8 minutes or until salmon flakes easily when tested with fork.

3. Whisk milk into flour in small bowl until smooth. Stir into saucepan. Cook until heated through.

Makes 8 servings

Last Look

While the philosophy behind oil-pulling is centuries old, the considerations for oil-pulling are ever going. Contemplate the advantages and disadvantages of oil-pulling and individual body and health stipulations. Choose wisely, practice (if you do) oil-pulling smartly and as always, check with dental and health care professionals before attempting any new routine.

Red onion and red bell pepper (with vitamins A and C), sautéed in delectable coconut oil, with green beans and fresh dill mixed with skinless salmon (with calcium, protein and vitamin D), milk (with vitamins A and D and protein) and wild rice (with B-vitamins) make a hearty one-dish meal that is great for the teeth, bones, and appetite!

A Natural Alternative

While coconuts are delicious and versatile and their meat, oil, and water do amazing things for our appearance and health, there are some other surprising and lesser-known ways that the coconut can be used to support a natural and healthful lifestyle.

Coconut products can act as household cleansers, lubricants and conditioners; shine jewelry, leather goods and shoes; remove rust; and are the basis for useful homemade items. They can even provide raw materials for various building and household goods.

Household Cleanser, Lubricant, and Conditioner

One of the concerns about household cleaners is that their chemicals are emitted into our homes and we are exposed to their ingredients. Instead, a growing number of people are interested in "green" cleaners, or products that are produced with biodegradable, natural, and nontoxic ingredients. Coconut and its by-products can claim all three attributes.

As a household cleanser, coconut oil can remove simple dirty marks from surfaces that can handle commercial cleansers. Of course, it is always sensible to try a test area first before wider application.

Coconut oil may grease hinges and small appliances as it gently removes rust and it may remove simple stains and condition wooden floors and moldings. Once applied, make sure to dry and buff the treated areas with a soft cloth and take care to walk on these parts carefully.

Cleanses and Conditions Household Items

Coconut oil can be used as a handy, inexpensive and natural household cleanser to clean brushes and remove chewing gum, crayon marks, and ink spills on clothing, furniture, or floors. This may take a few applications, drying and fluffing or buffing with a soft, dry cloth.

Coconut oil can be lightly melted, then applied with a clean, dry, and soft cloth to clean and add shine and protection to a host of natural household surfaces instead of using synthetic cleaners and conditioners. Follow with another dry buffing cloth. A little residue can be left behind for extra shine and conditioning. If anything adheres to the coconut-oil residue, then a simple rinse may be needed before using.

Cleanses and Smoothens Brushes

After paintbrushes are used and cleaned, they may become hardened—even if water-based paints are used. Coconut oil will keep paintbrushes supple and ready for use. Make sure that they are impeccably cleaned before applying so the paint is not activated.

Makeup Brush Cleaner

Rub warmed coconut oil on make up brushes and let set a few hours. Wash thoroughly and dry well with a clean, dry cloth. A little residue may be desirable to revitalize the brush hairs and for makeup application.

Removes Chewing Gum from Hair or Furniture

When coconut oil is applied to hardened chewing gum it may ease the adherence and make it easier to dislodge, without leaving behind any residual colors or stains.

Liberal amounts of coconut oil may be applied on to the chewing gum and left to remain for about two to five minutes. Then a soft, dry cloth can be used to dislodge the chewing gum and remove the residue. Depending upon the fabric and care directions, a mild soap may be used to remove any excess coconut oil. A clean, dry cloth can then be used to blot any extra coconut oil.

Coconut oil can also be used to remove labels or other sticky residue in a similar manner. Try it with labels that adhere to glass, plastic, wood, or other hard surfaces, but be sure to check the care instructions first.

Cleans Crayon Marks, Ink Spills, and Spots

Crayon marks, ink smears, smudges, and skid marks may be removed with coconut oil by using a clean cloth or soft brush. Once the coconut oil sets for a few minutes, it can then be removed with another dry, clean cloth.

Cleans Metal Items

Assorted metal items may benefit by a thin layer of coconut oil, including cars, cast iron equipment, decorative objects, hinges, kitchen appliances, lawn mowers, snow shovels, zippers, bike chains, and much more.

Maintains and Details Cars

Coconut oil adds a lustrous sheen to the dashboard or to leather car seats. Test a little first with a clean cloth and buff it dry with another clean, dry cloth since materials differ. Remember that the coconut oil residue may be slightly slippery when passengers use the seats. Coconut oil can also be used to buff out little exterior scratches with a dry, clean cloth or to remove bugs or sap off of a car's exterior; first letting it coat the exterior for a few moments before wiping clean and dry.

Lubricates Small Motors and Kitchen Appliances

A small amount of coconut oil can be used to lubricate small motors, such as those in blenders, food processors, hand mixers ,or juicers—much like it can be used to oil hinges. Make sure that there is little-to-no residue that can solidify and prevent normal operation of these small household items.

A thin layer that is carefully rubbed over the blades of kitchen appliances helps to keep them running smoothly. Be extra cautious to unplug the appliances first before application and to carefully wipe in one direction and away to help prevent any accidents.

Seasons Cast Iron Cooking Equipment

Cast iron cooking equipment is prized for its ability to conduct heat and transfer from the stovetop to the oven then the table. The process of seasoning cast iron cooking equipment involves coating it with a layer for protection and to act as a non-stick surface. Coconut oil is excellent for both of these purposes and can be used like other vegetable oils.

A generous amount of coconut oil can be applied to the inside of cast iron cooking equipment. It can then be placed in a 250 to 350 degree Fahrenheit oven for about an hour.

If the coconut oil smells or starts smoking then remove the cooking equipment and turn down the heat. When the oven cools, put the items back into the oven. A cookie sheet can also be placed under the items to prevent any coconut oil from spilling onto the oven floor.

Prevents Kitchen Items from Sticking

• Apply coconut oil in measuring cups or spoons before filling with sticky ingredients, such as honey or maple syrup.

• Rub the inside of plastic storage containers with a little coconut oil to prevent deeply-colored stains from gravies, soy sauce, tomato sauce or other highly-pigmented items.

• "Grease" the inside of cake pans or muffin tins with coconut oil before the batter is added to help easily remove baked goods. It is important to use a clean, dry cloth and apply a thin layer; then wipe off any extra coconut oil with another clean, dry cloth since any residue may smoke in the oven. Also, be careful when they are used as they might be slippery.

Once the cooking equipment is removed from the oven, any excess coconut oil can be wiped off with a clean, dry cloth and discarded. This process should be repeated a few times until the surfaces are functionally non-stick.

Maintains Lawn Mower Blades and Knives

A thin layer of coconut oil that is rubbed over clean lawn mower blades helps to prevent clumps of grass from sticking and jamming the lawn mower. Likewise, stained, dulled knives may be refreshed with a thin layer of coconut oil. As with the small appliances blades, stroke away and in one direction.

Slicks Snow Shovels

Sometimes snow and ice cling to shovels and other winter removal equipment. Once a thin layer of coconut oil is applied to this equipment, the snow or ice should be able to be removed more easily. This process may need to be repeated with on-going snow, ice and other weather issues.

Reduces Squeaky or Sticky Hinges

A little coconut oil may be all that is needed to reduce the stickiness or squeakiness in cabinets or door hinges.

Unzips Zippers and Greases Bike Chains

A thin layer of coconut oil can be applied to jammed bike chains or heavy-duty zippers. Coconut oil functions as a natural lubricant for bike chains and to keep zippers operating smoothly.

Just a little coconut oil that is applied to a jammed clothing zipper should help it to move easier or get back on track. Make sure that it is rubbed into both sides of the zipper before moving it and that any excess is removed so as not to damage garments or leather goods.

Reduces and Removes Rust

Rust is caused by the reaction of iron and oxygen in the presence of air or water. To remove rust, apply a thin layer of coconut oil over a rusty area. First rub a little coconut oil on metal objects, such as car accessories, outdoor metal furniture, silverware, or other metal items that are disposed to rusting to test the results. Then, apply just a thin layer of coconut oil with a soft, dry cloth and let it remain on the metal object for a few hours. The coconut oil can then be wiped or washed off with warm water depending upon the surface of the object and if there are any care instructions that advise otherwise. The object can be cleaned of any rusty residue and dried with a clean, dry cloth. Repeat the process if necessary. The improvement should be fairly immediate and provide longer-range protection.

Eliminates Soap Scum

Apply a thin layer coconut oil to soap scum in the bathtub or shower and let it remain about 10 to 20 minutes. Soap is alkaline and coconut oil (as are other oils) is acidic, so the coconut oil works to break down soap scum. Vinegar can be added to the coconut oil to increase its acidity or coconut oil can be mixed with baking soda into a paste. Dry the area with a clean, dry cloth and be careful to avoid slipping.

Polishes Metals

Coconut oil that is rubbed over clean metal with a soft cloth, left for a few moments, then buffed to a shine helps to restore the polished look of metal surfaces. Coconut oil is particularly useful for polishing bronze items.

Conditions Leather Chairs and Sofas

Rub a small amount of coconut oil into real leather chairs or sofas to soften and condition them. While a little residue can remain, too much may residue may transfer to clothing or cause slippage.

Cleans and Polishes Granite Surfaces

Apply coconut oil onto granite counter tops, tables or other stone surfaces to clean and remove dust, cover minor scratches, and shine. Like other applications, it is best to try a small area first.

While some granite is intended to shine, other granite surfaces are meant to be duller in appearance. The sheen may be able to be adjusted.

Many creams and polishes form a layer of synthetic chemicals to create sheen and coat surfaces. Coconut oil is absorbed into any cracks or crevices and may last longer. Plus, coconut oil lends a pleasant smell throughout the kitchen and the rest of the house.

Conditions Cutting Boards

Kitchen cutting boards should first be cleaned with a damp towel. Then they should be dried well before coconut oil is applied. A different soft cloth should be used to rub some coconut oil into the surface of the cutting board. After the cutting board absorbs the coconut oil for about 10 to 15 minutes, then another fresh, dry cloth should be used for buffing.

A little lemon essential oil or lemon juice can be added to the coconut oil first to remove any odors and to provide a pleasant lemon scent.

Shines Plant Leaves

Just a dab of coconut oil applied with a clean, dry cloth and gently rubbed across the surface of broad plant leaves helps them to look shiny and keeps them relatively dust-free. Repeat this process as needed. Some plant leaves do not thrive with a coating of any kind, so it is best to check with a nursery or plant care guide before application.

Shines Jewelry

Some types of jewelry can be polished with coconut oil, but it is best to check the care instructions first and try a little dab on the underside of the jewelry before possibly damaging. Bronze items may particularly benefit.

A dab of doconut oil is even handy for removing rings when they become too tight for the fingers.

Shines and Revitalizes Leather and Patent Leather Items

Rubbing coconut oil on leather or patent boots or shoes helps them to shine and revitalizes their overall appearance, including any buff or scratch marks. This process may need to be repeated over time. As with other leather goods, it is best to try a test area first before full application.

Deters Pests and Soothes Bites

As an insect repellent, coconut oil has many applications. Coconut oil can be mixed with essential oils such as citronella, peppermint, rosemary, or tea tree or herbs such as catnip, mint, or rosemary as a natural insect repellant to repel bees, flies, or gnats. Apply liberally. This mixture provides a safer alternative to some insect repellants and can usually be applied all over the body. If bitten, coconut oil dabbed directly onto a cleansed and sanitized bug bite might offer some relief.

Creates Useful Homemade Items

Items as simple as candles, laundry detergent, and play dough can be made with coconut oil. It is generally easy to use, inexpensive, natural, and perfumes the house, clothing, and hands with its attractive tropical coconut smell.

Turning a hard coconut shell into a bowl or makeshift musical instrument is also a creative use of the coconut.

Play Dough

Play dough is a popular childhood product that can be made with melted coconut oil, salt, flour, water, cream of tartar, and natural food coloring with this recipe:

1	**tablespoon coconut oil**
½	**cup salt**
1	**cup flour**
1	**cup water**
2	**tsp. cream of tartar**

Natural food coloring

1. In a large, heavy pot, melt 1 tablespoon coconut oil over low heat.

2. Gradually mix the next four ingredients into the melted coconut oil.

3. Stir until the mixture forms a ball.

4. Add the natural food coloring and mix well.

5. Remove from heat and cool before using.

6. Store in an airtight container.

Laundry Detergent

Melt pure soap, then mix with coconut oil and essential oils and add a little water. Pour this mixture into a container or mold to harden. It makes a non-toxic liquid or solid depending upon the amount of water that can be used as a laundry detergent to clean clothes. This combination should not be irritating nor affect fabrics, but is it best to try a little on a small patch of skin and item of clothing before applying. People who are prone to allergies and/or have sensitive skin may benefit from this use.

Serving Utensils

The hard, outside shells of coconuts can be cleaned well, dried, and prepped with coconut oil, then used as serving bowls for dried foods, such as chips or crackers. Make sure to clean these containers well after each use and prep with coconut oil again as needed.

Musical Instruments

Empty coconut shells can be turned on their cut ends and played as percussion instruments—much like they have been used around the world for centuries for musical entertainment. Even children can use coconut shells for simple drums that can be first decorated.

Scents

Mix coconut oil and essential oil in an oil diffuser to create economical, natural and inviting scents without artificial ingredients.

Aromatherapy

Add a few drops of comforting essential oil to warmed coconut oil. Daub on the back of the neck, the tip of the nose, on the chest, or on the temples. Try eucalyptus or peppermint essential oil for congestion or stress reduction, or for an upset stomach, try a citrus-based essential oil, such as lemon, lime, or orange.

Protecting Your Pet

The coconut's healing and protective properties don't just apply to you—they can help your pet as well! Coconut oil can be used to clean dog or cats' ears and to moisturize dry, cracked paw pads or noses. It can even be used to make homemade, natural treats for some pets. And coconut oil helps prevent cat litter from sticking to the bottom of a litter box when the box is rubbed with a thin layer.

Grooms Pets

Just like coconut oil is beneficial for human skin and hair, coconut oil contributes to the silky coats of dogs and cats. It can be added to pet shampoo or warmed by human hands and lightly massaged into a pet's coat.

Relieves Dry, Injured, or Sensitive Skin

Besides being delicious, nutritious, and soothing for pets, a small amount of coconut oil may be nurturing when it is applied to a pet's sensitive or injured skin. Coconut oil may help nourish dry, inflamed or irritated skin that results from allergens, chemicals, insect bites, or other causes.

Some examples follow:

• One-half teaspoon of coconut oil that is applied to cat's paws may smooth dryness. A similar amount that is applied to a cat's furry exterior may promote a shiny coat and reduce hairballs.

• A similar amount of coconut oil that is rubbed into a dog's paws may prevent or reduce cracked paw pads. Dog paws tend to be calloused, rough, tough and/or thickened to handle the dog's daily walks.

Both dogs and cats might enjoy the taste of coconut oil and lick their paws clean. This might lead to increased licking and soreness, so it is best to monitor the process. It is also wise to apply the coconut oil to a dog's paws outside and away from delicate carpets or floors.

• Some warm coconut oil may be rubbed onto a cat or dog's nose that is chronically dry or cracked. Beware that the tastiness of coconut oil may promote constant licking and may defeat the original purpose of lubricating the cracked skin. Keep trying, as the newness of this application may eventually dissipate.

• A little warm coconut oil may be used to clean a pet's ears. First, any dirt should be gently removed with a cotton ball or soft cloth. Then, a little warm coconut oil may be gently rubbed into the underside of the ears with another clean cotton ball or soft cloth. Make sure to remove any residue beyond a thin layer. While a dog's ear canal is in an L-shape, it is still advised not to insert anything too far inside of a dog's ears. The coconut oil may help to keep the skin's interior supple and reduce itching. It is best to check first with a veterinarian before application—especially for smaller dogs.

• Coconut oil may also be used for dental hygiene. Add a few drops of coconut oil on a soft toothbrush to keep a dog's teeth clean, its gums healthy, and its breath smelling pleasantly. While coconut oil is edible and there is little health risk if pets lick it off, there may be exceptions. As with other usages of coconut oil for animals, exercise caution.

Nourishes Pets and Supports Pet Health

Similar to humans, dogs and cats may benefit from coconut oil added to their diet. The pet maladies that seem to benefit the best from coconut-oil enhanced pet food are skin allergies, irritations or wounds and digestive upsets.

A veterinarian should be first consulted. Dogs over 40 pounds of weight may benefit by one-half to one tablespoon of coconut oil and dogs under 30 pound of weight may benefit by half this amount or less to help to improve their dry skin and promote a healthy coat. It is best to start with a few drops to about one-half teaspoon of warmed coconut oil added to food daily; watch for any reactions. It there is unusual stomach upset or other contraindications then cut back and contact a veterinarian if any ill effects continue.

The saturated fatty acids in coconut oil, particularly the medium-chain triglycerides, provide energy for pets as they do for humans. There is some debate about the use of medium-chain triglycerides in the diet of cats, so it is best to talk to a veterinarian before it is used.

Coconut water can be frozen into ice cube trays and coconut water cubes can be given to pets on hot days as a cool and tasty refresher.

Coconut oil and peanut butter can be blended with a little coconut water to thin, poured into ice cube trays and frozen. These coconut pet treats are cold, nutritious, and tasty especially during hot, dry summers.

Coconut Oil Dog Treats

½ cup coconut flour

½ cup fruit puree (applesauce, apricot or pear)

1 tablespoon honey

2 tablespoons coconut oil

3 tablespoons water*

1. Preheat oven to 350°F.

2. Line cookie sheet with parchment paper.

3. Combine all ingredients; mix well until smooth consistency. Add more water if needed.

4. Pinch small pieces of dough with fingers; roll into ½ to 1-inch balls.

5. Place uniformly on parchment paper, leaving room between each ball.

6. Bake for five minutes; turn once, then bake an additional five minutes. Cool on rack.

7. Store in refrigerator or freeze.

Putting It All Together

We've discussed the many ways that you can put the coconut to work for you, the ways it may benefit your heart and brain health, its cosmetic applications, and the ways it may be used in a natural lifestyle. No one food or material can be a miracle cure—but the coconut has many versatile applications.

So now that you know, where do you go from here?

Cooking with Coconut

With some ingenuity, the coconut can be used in a number of tasty and inspiring recipes. Simply start by substituting a cooking oil with coconut oil in equal amounts and notice how the recipe changes. It will likely perk up the flavor and lend a rich-tasting texture. Remember the subtle sweetness of coconut oil when it is added to savory foods. It could temper the taste or create a new flavor of its own. The other ingredients may have to be adjusted to compensate. When adding coconut oil to sweet ingredients it will likely increase the sweetness.

Make sure that the recipe is compatible for this change. The other ingredients may need adjustment.

Fresh coconut, coconut water and coconut milk have a wide range of culinary applications.

Coconuts provide the backbone flavor in many tropical recipes with southern Indian, Southeast Asian, African, and South American roots. Unless coconuts are toasted or kept very dry, coconuts tend to have a lasting flavor and chewy texture.

Flaked or grated coconut or coconut milk can be used in puddings, pies and cakes for taste, moisture, and texture; sprinkled over fruit or compotes; added to cookies, candies, and confections; blended into curries and sambals (curry accompaniments) and mixed into side dishes, soups, stews, and stir-fries to elevate simple proteins, starches, and vegetables into distinctive aromatic and appetizing complex dishes. Some of them appeared throughout this book, and we've included a few more here!

Banana Berry Coconut Milk Smoothie

1 cup unsweetened coconut milk

1 medium banana, peeled

1 cups berries (blueberries, raspberries and/or strawberries)

4 to 5 whole ice cubes

1 tablespoon coconut oil (optional)

Nutmeg (optional)

1. Place the first four ingredients into a blender.

2. Blend at low speed until smooth.

3. Dribble with coconut oil, if desired*.

4. Blend at medium speed until well blended.

5. Top with sprinkle of nutmeg, if desired.

Makes 2 cups

The coconut oil should be added slowly while the blender is running after the main ingredients are blended. This will ensure that it is evenly distributed. If the coconut oil is added sooner, then it might harden into little beads and prevent a smooth consistency.

Coconut Selection

Before you cook, you'll have to shop for your coconut or coconut byproducts. Here are some tips.

• The hard, green coconut shells are generally removed before coconuts are marketed. What remains are the smaller, rounded brown shell that are usually covered with brown and hairy fibers. The best seasons for purchasing coconuts are fall and winter.

• Select heavy coconuts that are filled with liquid which can be heard when a coconut is shaken. Whole coconuts are easier to crack and remove the coconut meat if that are frozen or heated first since the coconut becomes brittle. Whole coconuts last about 6 months at room temperature depending upon their degree of ripeness and about one month once refrigerated.

• It is best to avoid coconuts that are cracked, moldy or weep from the eye end. Once the coconut is cracked open, if the coconut is yellowed it is best to discard it since it is likely spoiled.

• Coconuts are also available processed in flaked, grated and shredded forms, unsweetened and sweetened and dry and moistened.

• Shredded coconut is found in cans and packages; coconut in cans is usually moister.

• Canned or dried coconut lasts about 18 months unopened and one month once opened and refrigerated.

Coconut Conversions

• One medium coconut yields about three to four cups of grated coconut meat.

• One 7-ounce bag of shredded coconut yields about three cups of shredded coconut.

• One 3 ½-ounce can of shredded coconut yields about ⅓ cups of shredded coconut.

Cracking Coconut

To crack a coconut, follow these steps:

1. Drive a long, thin spike though one of the coconut's three "eyes" that is located at one end of the coconut.

2. Drain the liquid and strain. It can be consumed or refrigerated.

3. Crack the nut with a hammer or other strong implement. You may want to cover the nut with a kitchen towel to prevent any flying pieces.

4. Continue to break the nut with the hammer or other strong implement until it splits into smaller pieces.

5. Carefully cut the white coconut "meat" away from the shell with a sharp knife. A kitchen towel may help to stabilize the larger pieces as they are cut.

6. If the coconut meat is cover with coconut debris, then gently rinse and pat dry with a clean, dry cloth.

7. Chop or grate the coconut meat with a sharp knife, box, or rotary grater or food processor.

8. Bag and refrigerate the chopped or grated coconut for up to five days.

Toasting Coconut

Spread a thin layer of flaked, grated or shredded coconut in a nonstick jellyroll pan. Bake at 350° F about 10 to 20 minutes or until lightly browned. Stir the coconut frequently as it browns very rapidly. Remove the jellyroll pan with the coconut from the oven and allow to cool. Refrigerate or wrap the coconut in freezer paper; leave some "head space" and freeze.

Personal Care

Because coconut oil is so economical and versatile, the use of coconut oil in personal care recipes holds a wealth of possibilities. Look for old apothecary-type recipes and substitute coconut oil (and maybe a little coconut water) for the fats in the recipes. Or add a little smidgeon of coconut oil to recipes for its richness and moisturizing potential. Make sure to use sterilized containers and clean hands or clean and dry cloths to ensure safety. And do refrigerate the finished products for safekeeping.

The coconut nourishes, cleaned, protected, and outfitted people around the world for centuries and still functions in these varied capacities today. Explore the vast range of practices that are outlined in this book and see what it may do for you!

No-bake Coconut Bites

2	old-fashioned oats
1½	cups coconut flakes
1	cup almond butter*
1	cup ground flaxseed**
⅔	cup honey
2	teaspoons vanilla

1. Place oats into bowl of food processor; process about 10 seconds or until flaked.

2. Combine remaining ingredients in large mixing bowl; mix with spatula or hands.

3. Refrigerate about 30 minutes.

4. Pinch dough; shape into 1-inch balls.

5. Place on waxed paper; refrigerate until slightly hardened.

6. Remove and place into food container; refrigerate or freeze.

*Peanut butter can be substituted if a peanut allergy is not an issue.

**Ground flaxseed is used because the seeds are hard to chew and swallow. Grinding makes the flaxseed easier to digest.